BE A
BETTER
RUNNER

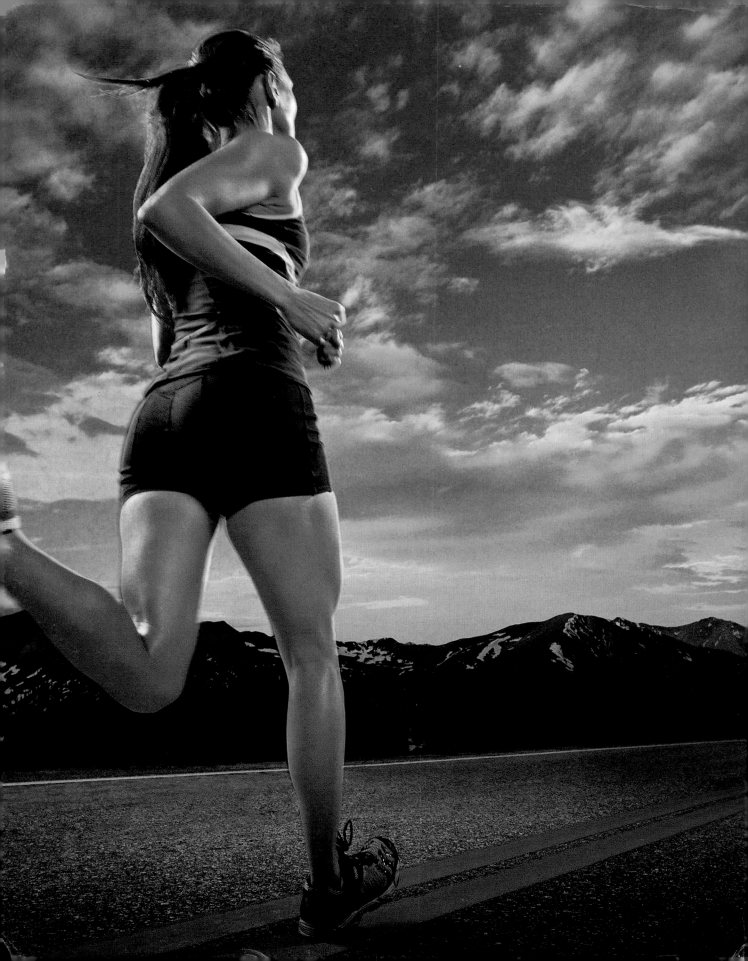

BE A BETTER RUNNER

REAL-WORLD, SCIENTIFICALLY PROVEN TRAINING TECHNIQUES THAT WILL DRAMATICALLY IMPROVE YOUR SPEED, ENDURANCE, AND INJURY RESISTANCE

SALLY EDWARDS
Ultra-marathoner, former master's world record holder in the Ironman Triathlon, and Triathlon Hall of Fame inductee

CARL FOSTER, PH.D., F.A.C.S.M.
Professor of Exercise and Sport Science, University of Wisconsin–La Crosse

ROY M. WALLACK
Los Angeles Times fitness columnist and author of *Run for Life*

First published in the USA in 2011 by
Fair Winds Press, a member of
Quayside Publishing Group
100 Cummings Center
Suite 406-L
Beverly, MA 01915-6101
www.fairwindspress.com

15 14 13 12 11   1 2 3 4 5

ISBN-13: 978-1-59233-424-7
ISBN-10: 1-59233-424-5

Library of Congress Cataloging-in-Publication Data available

Photography: Matthew Modoono

Printed and bound in China

The information in this book is for educational purposes only. It is not intended to replace the advice of a physician or medical practitioner. Please see your health-care provider before beginning any new health program.

>>> ACKNOWLEDGMENTS

Dr. Steven Seiler and Dr. Jonathan Esteve-Lanao, for the groundbreaking studies that helped identify the Black Hole.

Roy Wallack's Dedication: To Norman Wallack, possibly the coolest dad in the universe.

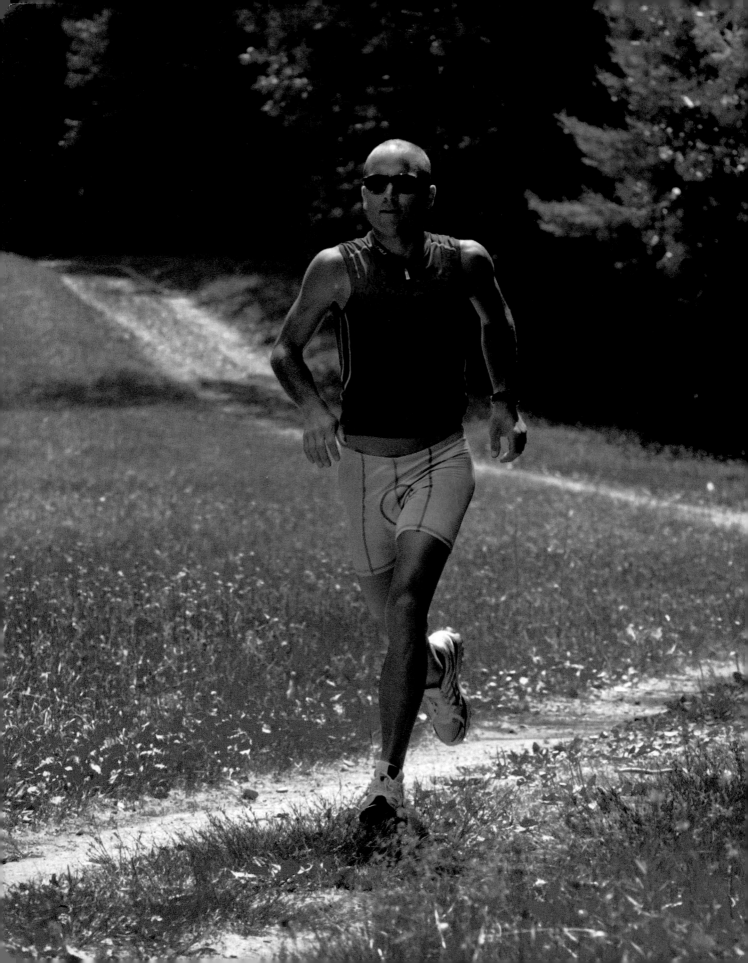

>>> CONTENTS

>>>

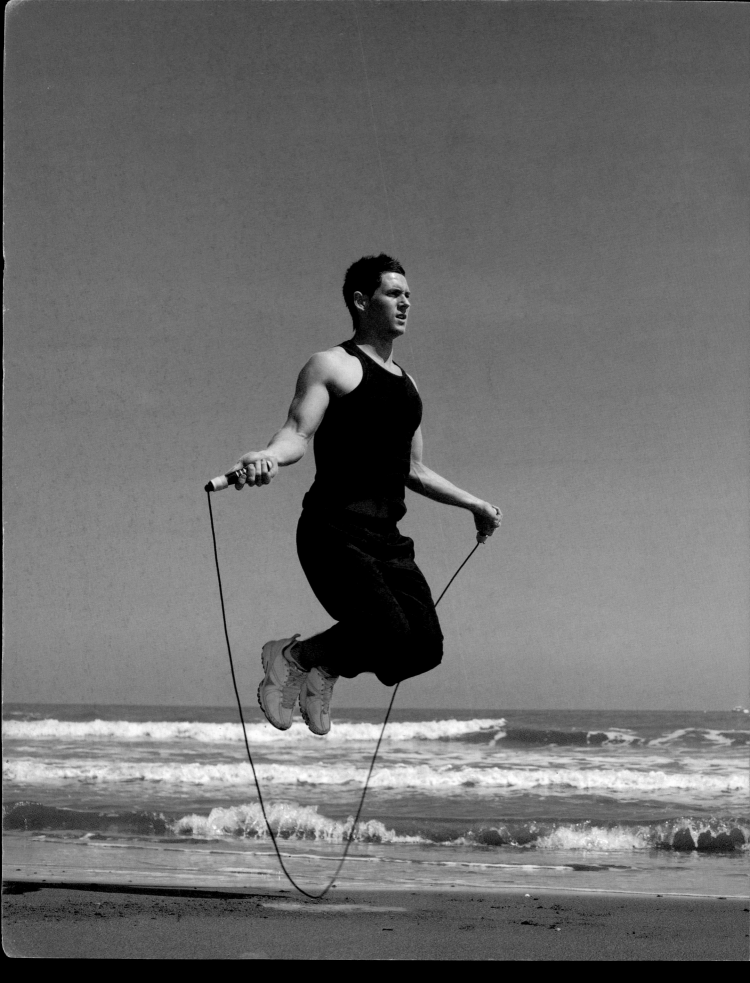

THROUGH THE CROWD, just as the clapping that filled the conference room began to die down, I saw Carl coming at me. "Of course, we've known all along that it's all true!" he said of the speech just delivered here at the annual meeting of the American College of Sports Medicine (ACSM) by Dr. Daniel Lieberman, a Harvard professor of evolutionary biology who discussed the research that underlies his theory that shoeless human hunters ran long distances in daily life for thousands of years before civilization began. "Everyone on this planet was born a runner!" he said.

"Yes," I responded. "Running is so enmeshed with our identity and history and survival that it's almost spiritual. It connects you with who you are. To not do it almost makes you less human in a way, doesn't it?"

Carl Foster, Ph.D., esteemed exercise physiologist and professor at the Department of Human Kinetics at the University of Wisconsin-La Crosse, nodded knowingly. "It was great to hear that what we've instinctively known about running can now be backed up by the facts," he said. "And you and I have been thinking about, and writing about, the hard facts about running for a long, long time, you know?"

Yes, I know. Carl and I have known each other since the mid-1990s, when we met for the first time at another ACSM meeting. As we like to say, we clicked right away because we started arguing within thirty seconds!

I favored heart rate as a way to measure performance. He favored RPE, the Rating of Perceived Exertion system of Gunnar Borg of Stockholm University. Both he and I are strong personalities, are highly competitive, and do not give an inch. I'd founded one of the world's biggest running shoe stores, Fleet Feet, and finished second in the 1981 Hawaii Ironman triathlon. He'd gone mano a mano with some of the world's top athletic theoreticians. He forced me to defend myself—and as anyone who knows me will tell you, I always defend myself.

I was right, he was wrong. My heart rate analysis was objective. His RPE, despite the numbers and regression analysis you might wring from it, was subjective. On top of that, I was arguably the expert on heart rate training—Carl even admitted that he'd read my heart rate book, the first of its kind on the then-new heart rate monitor and called it "quite bright." That made me glow, because it might as well have been a compliment from the mouth of God.

After all, even though Carl was wrong about heart rate versus RPE, he didn't just fall off the turnip truck. After doing his dissertation under the wing of academic and coaching legend Dr. Jack Daniels, Carl went on to establish himself as one of the world's foremost authorities in analyzing and quantifying athletic performance. And his curiosity was limitless. For years, he'd been studying everything from the VO_2 max of an Olympic 1,500-meter runner to the oxygen uptake of a cardiac patient trying to climb a flight of stairs. Carl's depth of knowledge in the field of running and athletic performance was legendary.

After we went back and forth for a while, I finally looked at him. "Carl, why are you wasting all your time talking to all these scientist geeks—and not the masses?" That stopped him cold. A light bulb turned on in his head. Right then, we agreed to start some projects together —beginning with some quantifiable studies of my heart rate zones methodology. Remember, it was still the early days of heart rate training. *Polar* had just come out with the heart rate monitor a few years before, and no one really understood it. Well, no one except for maybe a few people who had read my book.

I invited Carl to speak with me in 1993 at a workshop I organized at the Milwaukee Heart Institute. It was there that he suggested a way to use my Heart Zones Training System to accomplish the same task that researcher Eric Bannister had with his well-regarded Training Impulse (a.k.a. TRIMPS score), which quantified training load. We've been friends and working together ever since.

I've written twenty-two books, all on heart rate, running, and triathlons, but have been pestering Carl to coauthor a broad-based running and fitness book with me for at least ten years. I didn't find that any of the running books out there—even my own—really put all the up-to-date knowledge together: the new research about gait, the cutting-edge training regimens, or the quantifiable analyses Carl had been immersed in. And I didn't want this book to be limited to high-end super-athletes, but rather to be geared to beginners on up, those who are working up to their first 10Ks, as well as long-time veterans looking for a personal record (PR) in their age groups.

For a decade, Carl had been too busy to think about a book. But getting a dose of Lieberman's research that day in Seattle about how we humans were literally born to run seemed to turn him—and the running public—on. Career runners who, for decades, just went out and ran, giving no thought to scientific methods and techniques, were now actively seeking new information for the first time. And the general public was too: Stoked by the new findings and frightened by the growing awareness of dangers of sedentary lifestyles and the obesity crisis, everyone is hungering for new information like never before.

"We need to write this book now," Carl said. "It isn't just Lieberman. There's an explosion of new knowledge out there about fitness and training, and you and I are actually a big part of it. Between the two of us, we have eighty years of running and science experience. We've got cutting-edge knowledge we can bring to the table that people need to know—about heart rate training zones, body-type predisposition strategies, proper form, performance, and diet—that can help people tap into the joy of running. And now, they finally want it. Yes, I agree with you—we're obligated to do it."

Hence, nine months later, like the birth of a baby, we introduce you to this book, which presents the cutting edge of the sport, for beginners and veterans alike, right at your fingertips. Some of the highlights include:

- **Heart Zones Training:** Sally has updated her acclaimed, easy-to-follow, instantly effective Heart Zones Training methodology for more speed and safety. Heart Zones takes the guesswork out of training, works for all levels of runners, and provides you with opportunities to objectively measure how much work you are actually doing.

- **The Black Hole:** Carl teaches you how to identify this to-be-avoided training zone that has been implicated by new research conducted by his colleague from Norway, Stephen Seiler, Ph.D. An impediment to running progress and recovery, the Black Hole is one of the most valuable new concepts in running training.

- **Personalized training:** You will learn how to focus your training and goal setting on your specific body type and ability, including three field tests you can do.

- **Fast form:** Is there a universal running technique, a one-size-fits-all for foot strike, arm swing, and body rotation, as many now claim? Learn how to individualize it for you.

- **Real R&R:** Rest can supercharge you, but only if it's the right rest at the right time. Here's how to tell the difference between deep sleep and dumb sleep, and real rest and restlessness.

- **Mix it up:** You'll learn why cross-training activities such as cycling, swimming, rowing, elliptical training, and hiking are not just a fun break from running, but are absolutely critical to running better.

- **Why weights:** Running alone is not enough. We tell you why a strong, flexible core and breath control are the overlooked keys to strong running—and show you the workouts to get them.

- **Gas in the tank:** The right food at the right time will dictate your ability to go long and strong, manage your weight, and recover quickly from hard workouts.

- **Race-day primer:** Learn how to score your best time by tapping the science of race physiology, digestion, and calorie usage.

- **Barefoot running:** Adherents of this small but growing back-to-nature trend claim injury reduction and running longevity, but there are a lot of unknowns. Is it right for you all the time, occasionally, or never?

To help it all go down easy, this book is filled with vivid photos and illustrations, designed to leave you with impressions that you'll never forget through decades of happy, healthy running. Remember, we're in this for the long run!

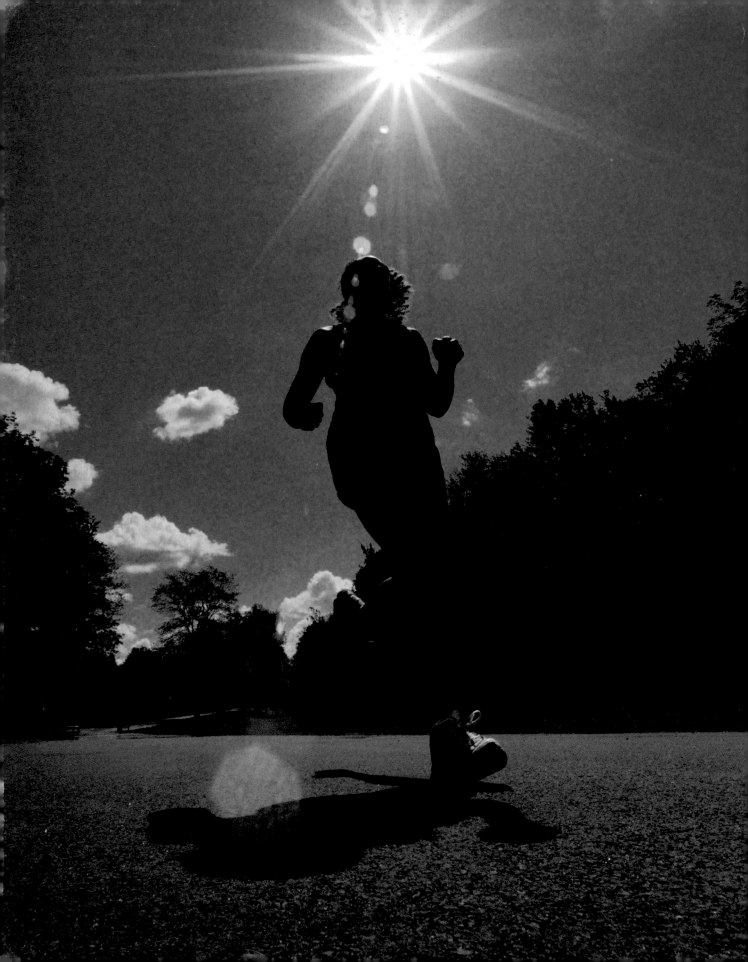

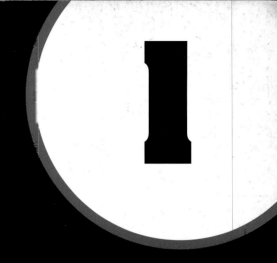

GET A HEAD START: A PREVIEW OF KEY CONCEPTS: HARD/EASY, THRESHOLD, AND THE BLACK HOLE

LIKE MANY SIMPLE THINGS, the plan you're going to read in this book is the culmination of a complicated journey. This book builds a highly individualized, easy-to-follow, time-efficient system for enhancing performance and lifelong fitness by combining years of cutting-edge research from top sports scientists and athletes with familiar concepts such as intervals, cross-training, recovery days, heart rate monitors, and better running form. It is centered on a patented training system called Heart Zones Training that fits on a pocket-sized chart, has a simplicity found nowhere else, and virtually guarantees success.

The plan is thoroughly logical, but there's a lot to digest here. That's why we are starting off by boiling down the main points of this book to a few pages that you can refer to as you read through it and implement the plan.

There is nothing subjective about this program. It's based on a careful, objective analysis of what has worked for top competitors, and then converts those principles into numbers that can be simply added up. Like clockwork, as your numbers grow, you'll safely ramp up your performance to new levels—if you stick to the plan, that is.

You see, the hardest part of this plan may be breaking your old habits. You know your daily run—that familiar, moderately hard-paced, thirty-minute route you've been doing five or six days a week for years, the one that gets you into your endorphin high? Say goodbye to it, or at least get used to seeing it a lot less. Although steady-state running does the trick for general fitness, it can also lead to repetitive-motion injuries, burnout, and gradual decline.

Our plan, different every day, does the opposite: It hardens and heals you, adds some challenges and variety that'll get you more excited about running, and very quickly makes you faster. It does this in two ways: It outlines the variation in intensity that the human body responds to by getting stronger, which we call Progressive Cross-Variability Training, and then teaches you how to precisely quantify the right intensities for you and schedule workout sessions to maximize their impact, which is accomplished through Heart Zones Training.

PROGRESSIVE CROSS-VARIABILITY TRAINING

As names go, this one is long but logical, as it replaces your old moderate-paced running with a variable plan that alternates hard and easy days, generously uses cross-training, and progressively pushes you harder over time. This sequence deliberately tears your muscles down, and then quickly builds them and your cardiovascular and fuel-burning systems back up, stronger than they were before. Over time, as you push even harder on the hard days, you'll get faster and fitter, lower your PR, move up in your age group, and even lose weight. Progressive Cross-Variability Training has one basic law and several supporting corollaries.

The one basic law is the hard-day/easy-day pattern: Always follow a hard running day with an easy workout. After all, that's how the body works: You stress your muscles beyond their comfort zone, and then give them time to heal so that they're even stronger. To make sure you stick to the hard/easy format, remember the following:

- Hard means hard. By hard runs, we mean intervals (from thirty-second all-out bursts to longer, faster-than-race-pace efforts) or runs that are longer than you are accustomed to.

- Easy means easy. On easy days, take the talk test. That means don't push it to the point at which you can't easily carry on a conversation as you work out. If you work too hard, you will not give your muscles time to rebuild to a stronger state. It also means "short." At the end of an easy day, you should feel fully rested and ready for the next hard day. If you aren't, take another easy day!

- Cross-train after every run, and don't run two days straight. All running, easy or hard, can be hard on the body. So, on the day after a run, go for an easy bike, swim, paddle, elliptical, or row, or don't work out at all. If you are strictly a runner (not a triathlete), there is generally no reason to do a hard cross-training day—unless you have an injury that prevents you from running but allows pain-free cross-training.

- Avoid the Black Hole (moderately hard running). Training at an in-between pace is no good because it is too hard to allow you to go as long as you should to improve your endurance and too easy to force the cardiovascular adaptations that come with high-intensity training. A key job of the Heart Zones Training System is to identify this Black Hole numerically via heart rate so that you can stay out of it.

- To get race-ready, ramp up the hard days. Make the hard days progressively harder to be at your best on race day. The body will respond to the additional stimulus.

HEART ZONES TRAINING SYSTEM

Good accounting is the key to making Progressive Cross-Variability Training work. After all, what good is asking you to do "hard" days and "easy" days if you don't know how to measure what is hard and easy? Before the heart rate monitor came along, you had to hire a coach with a stopwatch and clipboard who would carefully plan and monitor your workouts, and bark instructions at you from the infield of a high school track. But with the advent of the heart rate monitor, GPS, and speed and distance monitors, we have remarkably accurate technologies to keep you in touch with your body and allow you to coach yourself.

With good numbers in hand, you need a program to help make sense of them. That program, refined since the mid-1990s and now patented, is Heart Zones Training (HZT), which converts your complex heart rate data into a simple action plan for improvement.

Here's how it works. Heart Zones Training sets up five training zones based on heart rate. On a chart, the zones range from low to high heart rate:

- **Zone 1 (blue):** easy aerobic
- **Zone 2 (green):** moderate aerobic
- **Zone 3 (yellow):** hard aerobic
- **Zone 4 (orange):** extreme aerobic
- **Zone 5 (red):** unsustainable

In Zone 1, the heart rate range might be 90 beats per minute (bpm) to 100 bpm. Zone 2 might be 100 bpm to 120 bpm. Zone 5 might be 150-plus bpm. Zone 5 is red for a good reason: You're going anaerobic, literally redlining it.

The heart rate zones will have different ranges for everyone, since everyone's fitness and physiology is different. To set up your custom zones, you first have to find an anchor point to base them on: your threshold heart rate.

Threshold is a key concept mentioned again and again in this book, so get comfortable with it. Threshold is the point where you are running hard enough that your body begins to lose the battle to maintain homeostasis (or an internal equilibrium) and begins to tell you to slow down. When you cross over this intensity level, the effort is no longer sustainable "forever." For instance, you could be tooling along just fine at a heart rate of 140, 145, or 150 bpm, easily holding a conversation with your running partner, but when you speed up a bit more and raise your pulse to 155 bpm, your breathing suddenly gets harder and you find it more difficult to talk. If you had a lactate analyzer, you would observe that you are suddenly accumulating lactate in your blood. That's your threshold.

Threshold is technically a crossover point—when you cross over from a Zone 4 pace, where you can keep running all day (like at a marathon), to the faster, more stressful Zone 5 pace, where breathing gets harder and you can't tolerate more than twenty to sixty minutes, depending on your current level of run fitness, until you have to slow down. On the chart, you'll see that threshold is the line between Zone 4 and Zone 5. A fairly accurate and simple way to identify your threshold even without looking at the chart or a heart rate monitor is through the talk test: When it suddenly becomes hard to talk comfortably, you're at threshold.

Why is threshold important? Go back to the basic rule of Progressive Cross-Variability Training: If you want to get fitter, you have to do some of your runs fast—and that means at a pace beyond threshold. But how fast? Does that mean your fast runs can be at any speed, as long as it is above the threshold line? The answer is no.

It turns out that very fast runs are good for you—and that moderately fast runs (those just above threshold, in the Black Hole) are not. That's because Black Hole runs are too slow to cause enough stress to make your body want to strengthen itself, and too fast to allow you to go long enough to improve your endurance. Studies of top runners find that they (by design or not) minimize their time in the Black Hole.

How fast is the Black Hole? In terms of pace, heart rate, and the Heart Zones chart, the Black Hole is actually a very narrow band. It starts at threshold, right as you enter Zone 5, and goes about 5 percent higher. So, if your threshold heart rate is 150 bpm, your Black Hole would extend from 150 to 157 bpm. That means if you really want to improve, your fast runs should roughly start at a second threshold: 158 bpm.

In the Heart Zones system, there are actually two thresholds: The first threshold line is known as T_1 and the second threshold line is T_2. Therefore, your goal with the training described in this book boils down to this: Stay above T_2 and stay below T_1. Stay out of the Black Hole. (Or, in terms of the Heart Zones chart, stay out of Zone 5a, the first part of Zone 5, which you will see is divided into three sections, 5a, 5b, and 5c.)

The Black Hole is only five to ten heartbeats per minute wide, depending on your fitness, but staying out of it will not be as easy as it sounds, because it turns out that most people love to run there. Why? Well, the Black Hole is just hard enough that it makes them feel like they are doing themselves some good. Run in the Black Hole all the time, as most people do, and you end up tired, but no faster.

Your heart rate monitor is an invaluable tool in the Heart Zones system because, besides being interesting and fun, it gives you real numbers to attach to T_1, T_2, and the Black Hole.

Keep in mind that those numbers will increase over time as your fitness improves—which is a big advantage of Heart Zones over other systems. It's dynamic; it accurately reflects you as you are now, and it changes as you do.

THE BEST OF THE REST

The faster running sessions, measurable methodology, and better overall conditioning that this book's key chapters promote support and enhance the effect of the book's other sections.

- **Form:** Hard running helps teach you a more natural, injury-resilient form (see Chapter 10), which, although different for everyone and hard to change, includes a more vertical arm swing and some footstrike changes. Also included is an analysis of barefoot running and its impact on form and injuries.
- **Cross-training:** Unlike most running books, this program sees the integration of cross-training activities (see Chapter 4) as essential components of effective running.
- **Goal setting:** The sudden gains in performance will allow you to set more challenging goals (see Chapter 8), which you can set your mind to in the newfangled, old-fashioned way: by writing them down.
- **Diet:** The interval training advocated here will raise your metabolism for as much as twenty-four hours and burn more fat, resulting in significant weight loss when combined with a sensible eating plan (see Chapter 12).
- **Safety:** It's a jungle out there. All your effort to stay injury-free by honoring the easy days will be for naught if you don't observe the must-read safety rules in Chapter 13.

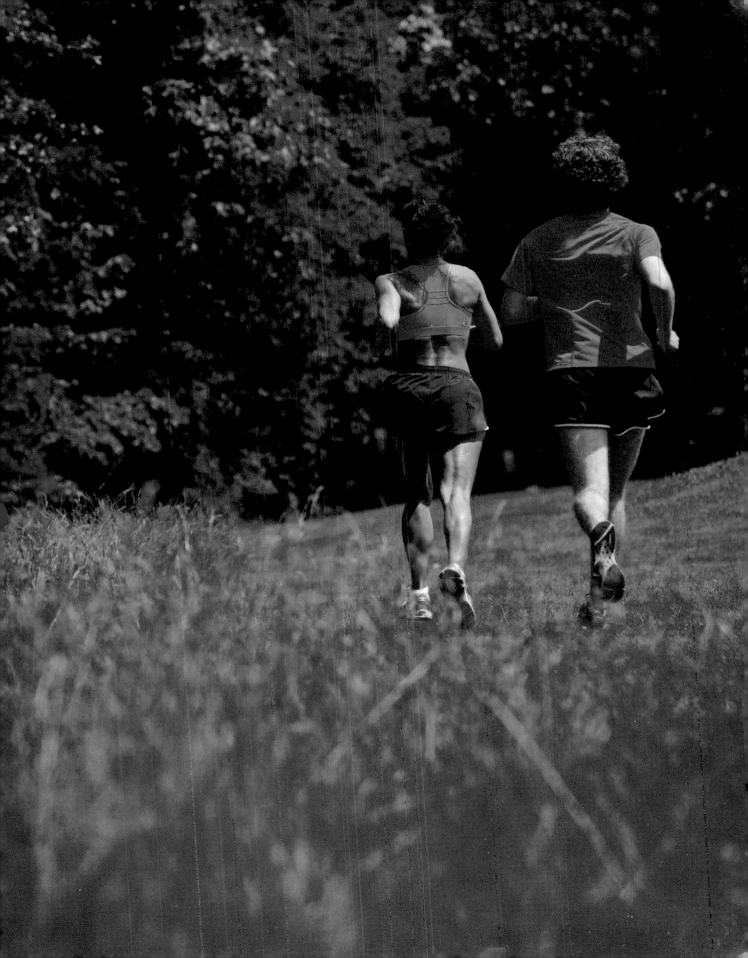

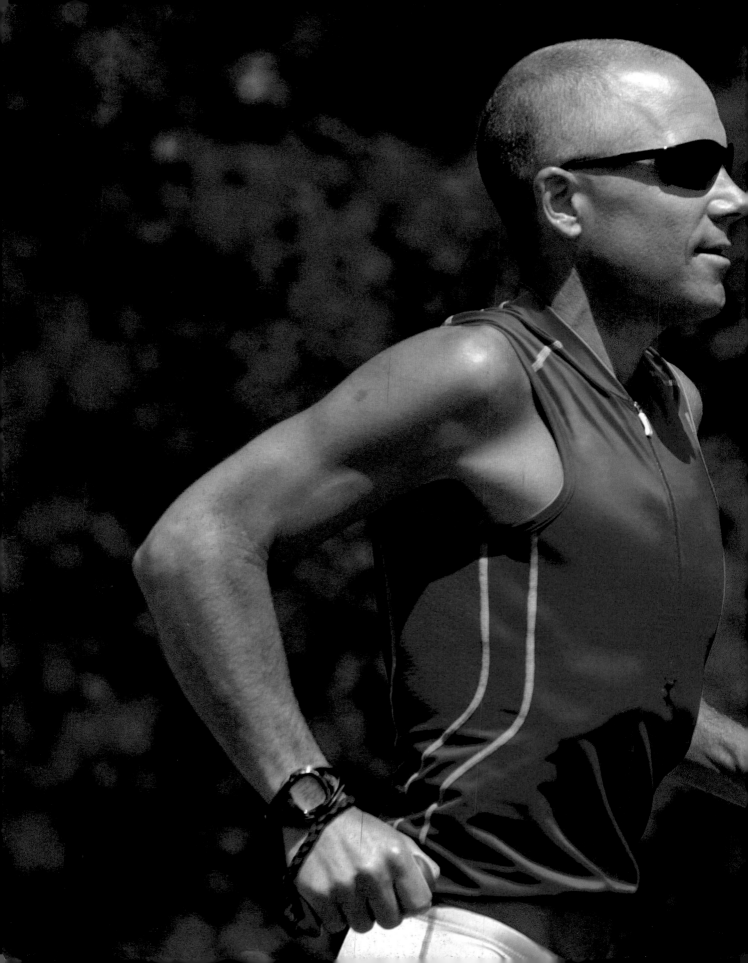

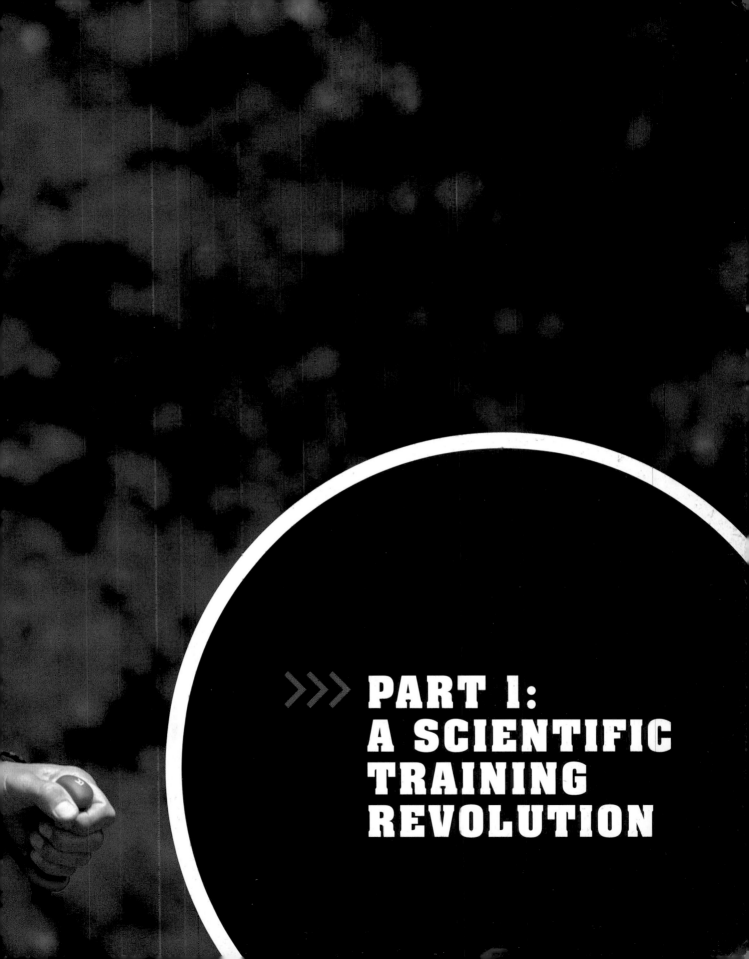

PART 1:
A SCIENTIFIC TRAINING REVOLUTION

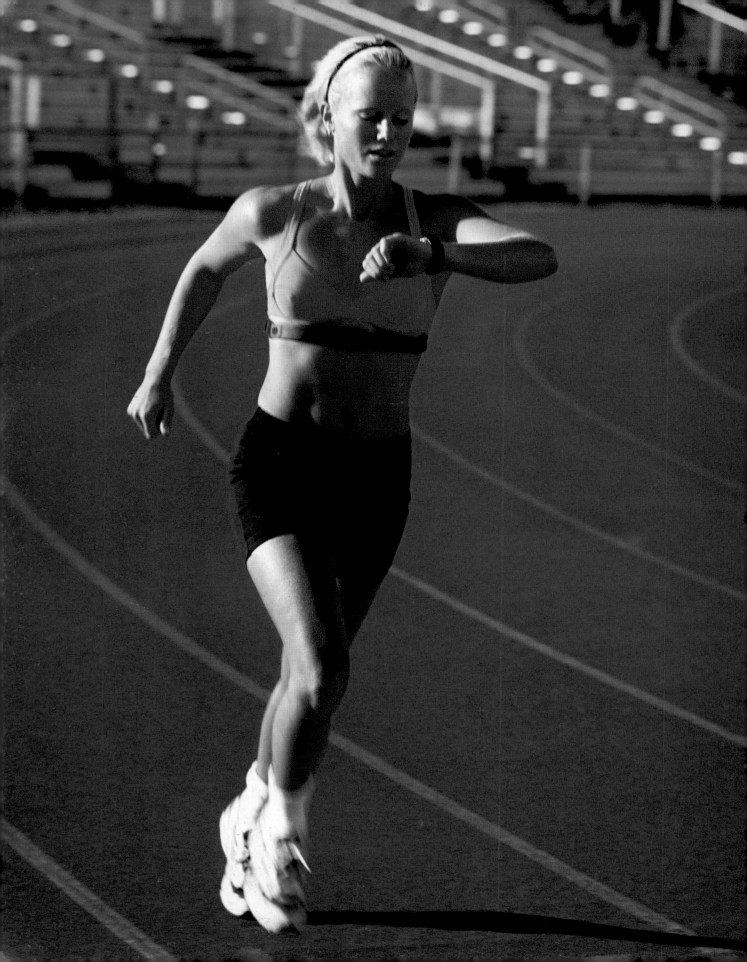

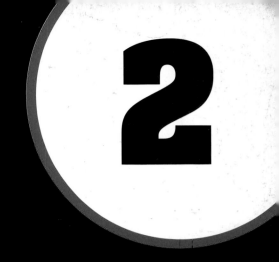

YOUR HEART RATE:
THE ULTIMATE TRAINING TOOL

I CRINGE A LITTLE BIT WHEN I hear coaches say they devise unique programs for every one of their athletes. True, everybody has unique responses to training stimuli. But that kind of personalization is simply not practical for the millions of runners who don't have the money or time for their own personal coaching guru. That's why, early in my running career, I started trying to devise a simple, universal grading system that would allow everyone to measure and plan their own workouts. After all, the first step in figuring out what kind of training works for you is being able to accurately assign values to what you did. After years of tinkering with technology and attending medical science conferences, I've assembled what I think is the world's most logical and easiest-to-use training scorecard: The Heart Zones Training System. Although it may look complex at first glance, Heart Zones is so simple and effective that you'll wonder how you ran without it, because it allows you to know exactly how hard and how easy you are working out.

THE HEART ZONES TRAINING (HZT) SYSTEM

Before I get into the detailed nitty-gritty, here's how it works, in a nutshell:

- **Objective scoring:** The HZT System is a great way to plan a training schedule because it is the first system that lets you objectively quantify your workouts. Based on how intense and how long you ran, you get Heart Zones Training Points (HZT Points). You can say, "I'm going to do a hard workout today of 50 HZT Points," and do exactly that. You can then follow that with an easier recovery workout that is valued at, say, 30 points. This also allows you to add your weeks up. As you gear up for a race, you can objectively plan and execute harder and harder weeks. There is no guessing; with Heart Zones, you know exactly how hard or how easy you are working out.

- **Easy setup:** The Heart Zones system uses a heart rate monitor to set up five distinct training zones, easy through hard. Each zone is a heart rate range: The easy zone might be from 100 beats per minute (bpm) to 120 bpm. The hard zone might be 150 to 160 bpm. Each zone is color-keyed blue, green, yellow, orange, or red, with blue being easiest and red being hardest.

- **Customizable:** The beats-per-minute limits of each zone will be different for every person, because they are based on your threshold heart rate. As you run faster, your heart rate gradually rises in order to pump more blood, which is filled with nutrients and oxygen, to your harder-working muscles. At a certain heart rate, you cross over a threshold where your ability to work almost indefinitely is exceeded (if you could take a blood sample at this point, you would also see that you are beginning to accumulate lactate in your blood). At threshold, or T_1, you start to feel that it is much harder to breathe and hold a conversation. In fact, a pretty accurate way to identify your threshold is through a talk test: When it suddenly is hard to talk, you're at threshold.

This threshold is now your reference point. All of the beats-per-minute limits of your five Heart Zones will be based on your heart rate at threshold, which could be 140, 150, 160, or somewhere in between, depending upon your fitness level. Your threshold will rise as your fitness improves, which is one reason it is such an accurate marker to use.

On the Heart Zones chart, threshold is the border between Zones 4 and 5, the orange zone and the red zone. Think of it as the dividing line between a serious but steady run and a hard run. Below that line are easier runs that give you moderate fitness. Above that line, it gets harder, which is good because going hard is one of the things you have to do to improve.

Now that you have a basic understanding of the Heart Zones system, you're ready for the details. Here's the story of how I came up with it, some technical background and history of training in general and Heart Zones in particular, and information about how to use the system to become a better runner.

A UNIVERSAL TRAINING SYSTEM: HEART ZONES TRAINING

I knew that the heart rate monitor could bring about a revolution in training if I could just figure out the application—how to use it as a way to train better than ever before. It could be a competitive weapon; those who used one would do better than those who ignored the application of technology to running. Now, with this real-time data, all I needed was a program that could use the data to systematize the training program.

That's when I decided to develop a universal training system based on zones, which I eventually dubbed "Heart Zones Training." As the name indicates, it uses the cardiac muscle (heart), sets up intensity ranges (zones), and works for those who exercise with a goal (training). You design your running program around different levels of heart rate intensity zones—an easy-effort zone with a low heart rate, a moderate-effort zone with a medium heart rate, and a hard-effort zone with a high heart rate.

I determined that a five-zone system was ideal for a lot of reasons. The primary reason for zone running is that it matches physiological changes or responses in your body to changes in intensity or effort. The five cardiac zones range from "easy" to "all-out." Mimicking the traditional way a coach might have you do a workout, you could design programs in which, say, you started off with five minutes warming up in Zones 1 and 2, the low heart rate zones; ten minutes cruising in Zone 3, the moderate heart rate zone; pushing it for several minutes into Zones 4 and 5, the high, hot zones, for speedwork and hard hill efforts; and then dropping back to Zone 3 for relief, and so on.

To make the Heart Zones Training System easy to understand visually, I give each zone a color:
- **Zone 1 (blue):** easy aerobic
- **Zone 2 (green):** moderate aerobic
- **Zone 3 (yellow):** hard aerobic
- **Zone 4 (orange):** extreme aerobic
- **Zone 5 (red):** unsustainable

To make the Heart Zones Training System easier to understand, I give each zone a name:
- **Zone 1 (blue):** the healthy heart zone
- **Zone 2 (green):** the temperate zone
- **Zone 3 (yellow):** the aerobic zone
- **Zone 4 (orange):** the threshold zone
- **Zone 5 (red):** the all-out red line zone

Creating a zone-training methodology actually was the easy part. The big challenge now was figuring out how to assign specific heart rate numbers to the zones, and where to draw the lines between the zones in a way that people would feel was meaningful, not arbitrary. That would be further complicated by the fact that everybody is different. A heart rate that is too high for one person might be too low for another person.

How to build a universal training system that was based on the Heart Zones Training methodology and applied to everybody; a universal system that worked for every sport activity; and a universal system for every gender, age, size, and interest level: That was the tough part.

And that was my challenge. As you'll see, it took a lot of learning about how the exercising body works—and a huge assist from my friend and coauthor, Carl Foster—to build a universal training system that I think is as useful and logical as anything ever developed. And it is one that works for everybody, for every heart, and for every step that is run.

SETTLING ON AN EASY-TO-USE ANCHOR POINT: THRESHOLD HEART RATE

Given that the heart rate monitor was such an efficient and relatively inexpensive tool, the first step to building a heart rate training system that works for everybody was to decide on a point of reference expressed in beats per minute (bpm) to which we can anchor the five heart zones. This anchor point had to be a physiological biomarker—a change in the body that was brought about by the changes in your workout effort (such as increase in speed).

Because our body undergoes a host of changes as we ramp up our training—it uses more muscles, increases breathing rate, heats up and sweats more, and taps different fuels—we have several biomarker anchor points to choose from. The trouble is that not all of these potential anchor points are practical for average people because they are hard to measure, require expensive equipment, require that you be in a laboratory, or all of the above. But they are good to briefly review because they all contribute to the system we finally settled on.

- Lactate threshold, the heart rate at which concentrations of lactate in the blood abruptly rise, requires you (usually while running on a treadmill) to prick your finger or earlobe to get drops of blood to feed into a blood-lactate analyzer. The testing is expensive, messy, painful, and complicated.

(continued on page 28)

It Started with a Heart Rate Monitor

My journey to find a universal training system began when I literally followed my heart.

When I bought my first Polar heart rate monitor in the early 1980s, I fell in love with it. It was primitive—hard-wired to a small box that I wore on my chest without a watch, with the heart rate data shown on a small display at the top. Several years later, I purchased one of the first wireless heart rate monitors, the Polar Vantage XL, for $400, a lot of money for a personal training tool that I knew little about. In 1984, I used it to train to quality—at age thirty-seven—for the first-ever women's Olympic marathon trials. To qualify to be one of the top 200 women in the United States to participate in the trials, I ran a 2:51 marathon—about twenty minutes behind Joan Benoit, who went on to win the trials. Being just past my prime at the time, I was very proud just to run in this historic event and to celebrate Joan's great victory at the Olympic Games in Los Angeles a few months later.

That was twenty-five years ago. Then, as today, I was convinced that everyone who does cardio-vascular exercise should be doing so with a heart rate monitor. I thought a heart rate monitor was the greatest thing in the world for so many reasons. I was so sure of it that I soon wrote the first book on heart rate training, titled *The Heart Rate Monitor Book.*

The book with the title that matched the device sold hundreds of thousands of copies, which further convinced me that, yes, someday everyone is going to run using this cool tool—the heart rate monitor.

I was dead wrong.

Although sales of heart rate monitors in Fleet Feet Sports, the chain of running stores that I co-founded, were brisk, so were returns. It turns out that hardly anyone knew what to do with this cool new training tool or what the numerical data meant. I loved knowing my heart rate while running, but the other runners seemed confused. So, I tried to think of a way to turn heart rate monitors into an understandable, usable, and motivational device for runners.

After all, using the heart rate monitor to tell you how much real work you're doing was a convenient and thoroughly objective way to quantify your run workouts. You could compare one day's workout to another, build a training program, use it to measure performance increases (and yes, decreases too), and objectively gauge whether what you were doing was yielding results.

Before the heart rate monitor, all runners guessed at how hard they were running, or their level of running intensity. To get any kind of handle of how your training translated to effort and to performance, you needed to have a coach with a clipboard, shouting out your minutes per mile (or meter) and writing down your split-times. This was years before the advent of the speed and distance monitors that used GPS or accelerometer technology that we have today.

With the heart rate monitor, for the first time in history you could begin to coach yourself—and probably do it more accurately—because you had real-time numbers about how hard or easy you were training. Coaches didn't have this—they didn't know the response to the effort you were exerting. This new device—a transmitter belt worn around your chest and wrist-top computer (the watch)—could serve as your coach and your guide. Once you learned how to program it, you could even set it to beep when you needed to increase your speed or slow down to meet your training goals. Mixing this data about your effort with a little understanding of cardio training, you could then interpret the data to show you how much volume coupled with the quantity of training make you faster, how much gets you injured, and in general, how much training (dosage) it takes for you to achieve your goals.

Bottom line: Now you could measure one of the all-important keys to successful running—your training load, or how much you actually work out.

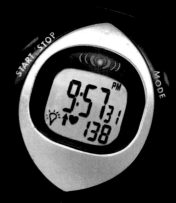

The Blink Heart Rate Monitor

- Ventilatory threshold is the heart rate at which there is a shift in the relative amount of breathing you have to do. Measuring ventilatory threshold requires a complicated, expensive metabolic cart (a.k.a. respiratory gas analyzer) that includes a breathing tube, face mask, wires, and black box (a breath analyzer).
- VO_2 max (maximum oxygen consumption), a reference standard since the early 1900s and considered by many exercise scientists to be the gold standard in fitness testing, is a measurement of your aerobic capacity. Usually expressed as the oxygen per kilogram of body weight per minute (ml/kg/min), it measures the amount of oxygen that you can consume at rest and during all-out exercise, adjusted for body weight.

Because your VO_2 max will change as you get more or less fit (a hypothetical unfit woman with a VO_2 max of 20 ml/kg/min could well improve to 30 ml/kg/min with a couple of months of serious training), VO_2 max is a good anchor to use with training zones. The trouble is that, like ventilatory threshold, it requires a metabolic cart when you run. That's just not practical.

That leaves us with two potential markers, maximum heart rate and threshold, both of which can be measured easily with simple heart rate monitors. Carl and I prefer to use threshold heart rate as an anchor point because it more accurately reflects your changes in fitness since it is a dynamic measurement. It changes as you improve. By comparison, maximum heart rate is static (fixed). But before I get into threshold, let me briefly explain the maximum heart rate system so that you know the differences.

- Maximum heart rate is the highest heart rate that you can produce when you reach the point of complete exhaustion during an all-out effort, when you simply can't go any faster or at a higher intensity. It is based on your genetic makeup and your sport activity. Running, for example, generally gives you a higher maximum than swimming, often by as much as 25–30 bpm. Maximums might be 200 bpm in a forty-five-year-old man or woman, or 175 bpm in a twenty-five-year-old man or woman. Similarly, two individuals of the same age can have maximum heart rates that differ from each other by as much as 40 or 50 bpm. The same is true of threshold heart rate numbers—but we'll get to that in a minute.

Unfortunately, maximum heart rate is more or less static, changing as slowly as a glacier in a fit population. It doesn't change much with fitness and decreases slowly with age.

Incidentally, you probably have heard of the common "220 minus your age" formula that many people use to determine maximum heart rate, but be aware that it is a creation more of convenience than of science, and that there is no equation to really accurately calculate your maximum heart rate.

Moreover, the maximum heart rate system, which we used successfully for many years until better evidence became available, sticks with its calculations regardless of the person's changing fitness levels, which is unrealistic.

That leaves us with the dynamic, fitness-influenced anchor point that we prefer: threshold heart rate. Don't confuse this with the previously mentioned thresholds, lactate and ventilatory; it's a broader measure that encompasses those thresholds. Threshold heart rate is a lower rate than maximum heart rate, and also very different for everyone, based on numerous factors. To understand the concept, think of threshold as a crossover point, the moment in your running where pushing harder will raise your heart rate enough to make it literally cross over into a new workout zone. It's like opening the door into a new room, a room that you just can't stay in for very long. As a result, in that new room, that new zone, different things will happen to you physiologically than happened before.

THE PHYSIOLOGY BEHIND THRESHOLD HEART RATE

The threshold system actually uses two different physiologic thresholds (and the heart rates associated with them), conveniently called T_1 and T_2—threshold 1 and threshold 2. In the laboratory, they are related to the ventilatory and respiratory compensation thresholds, which require technical expertise to measure. T_1 and T_2 are also related to blood lactate concentrations:

- T_1 is the lactate threshold, the heart rate at which the concentration of lactate in the blood makes its first real spike over its concentration at rest.
- T_2 is the point at which lactate begins to increase rapidly to several times its at-rest concentration.

T_1, also known as the "low threshold," is the heart rate at which you cross over from an intensity that is sustainable for a long time into a zone that you can sustain for only about twenty to sixty minutes—unless you are highly fit, in which case you can run a marathon at this pace.. So, T_1 is when the effort when it first begins to get hard: Your breathing rate increases and your sense of effort is that "this is beginning to get tougher and I better pay attention." Historically, this point has been referred to as both the "aerobic threshold" and the "anaerobic threshold," which makes it confusing; hence our use of T_1.

It is also the pace where you can talk comfortably. In addition, this is the point where you often turn to your running partner and say something to the effect of "If we're going to keep talking, we have to slow down." For a runner, the T_1 biomarker refers to your sustainable running pace or exercise capacity. "Sustainable" means your ability to continue exercising at the low threshold is mostly limited by the amount of muscle fuel, or glycogen, that you have saved up in your legs. For most reasonably well-trained people, this is two to three hours.

T_2, the second or "high" threshold, is also very distinct. It's like hitting one of those moments where you think, "I can't do this for more than ten to twenty minutes because it is so hard that I am on course for disaster, so I better either slow down or get to the finish line soon." Historically, this transition point has been referred to as the anaerobic threshold. When you cross over into this zone, conversation ceases, except for the gasping of single words, usually not-so-polite words.

Where do you find T_1 and T_2 on the five-zone Heart Zones Threshold Heart Rate chart? Low threshold occurs at the top of threshold Zone 4 and the bottom of threshold Zone 5. On the chart on page 30, it is depicted by a horizontal line separating the orange and red zones, marked with the words "low threshold." This horizontal gray line—the heart rate—is where you make the transition between fully sustainable effort and less sustainable effort. At the high-threshold point, you make the transition from less sustainable effort into only briefly sustainable effort.

The point at which ventilation and lactate are entering the realm of nonlinear increases is still a point where heart rate is increasing in a linear way. Thus, you can use your heart rate as a very convenient biomarker of this threshold point: The number at the point of the first threshold is your current anchor point, your current heart rate at low-threshold fitness. From now on, everything you do will be based on the heart rate at this 100 percent anchor point.

As for T_2, notice that everything above the low-threshold anchor point is Zone 5, which is colored red. That was not a random choice of colors. Because when you are above low threshold, you are literally redlining it. Within Zone 5, you find T_2: high threshold.

In a nutshell, then, here is your new running strategy: On different days, you train in different zones to get different benefits. For example, the day after a race, I like to do some easy running, so I set my heart rate monitor for Zone 2 which is 70 percent to 80 percent of my low threshold, and I take it slow and have a short workout. Many people call this a "recovery day" or a "Zone 2 day." On a fast training day, when I am doing my speed training, I might do medium-length interval training which would be track repeats of 0.5 miles (1 km) to 1 mile (2 km) in Zone 5a, or 100 percent to 105 percent of my low-threshold anchor heart rate number. Here's what it looks like for me:

SALLY'S RUNNING ZONES	FLOOR (BPM)	CEILING (BPM)
Zone 5a	140	147
Low Threshold 140 (bpm)		
Zone 4	126	140
Zone 3	112	126
Zone 2	98	112

When you cross over the heart rate level of T_1, one of many things that change is your metabolism (energy requirements). Low threshold, the first threshold, rests on the Heart Zones chart at the heart rate level between Zones 4 and 5a, and that is considered your 100 percent and the anchor point from which all the zones will be established. How do you attach a heart rate to it?

Remember, your T_1, your first threshold, is unique to you and principally to the unique elements of your metabolism. Whether it is 120, 150, or 180 bpm, your heart rate at T_1 is remarkably constant. Accordingly, we'll set up the five heart zones based on that anchor point.

To approximate your T_1, you don't need sophisticated, expensive instruments—just the heart rate monitor and your mouth. This method, developed by Carl, is called the threshold talk test.

FINDING YOUR T_1 WITH THE THRESHOLD TALK TEST

Carl Foster, Ph.D., is a past president of the American College of Sports Medicine and a professor at University of Wisconsin-La Crosse. One of his lines of work came in the practical application of Rating of Perceived Exertion (RPE). Combining RPE and a heart rate monitor, he created a way to score exercise bouts that combined intensity and duration. In other research, he adapted the idea that the talk test is uniquely related to correct training intensity and then created a more accurate threshold talk test, which has been validated in several peer-reviewed published articles.

How accurate is this simple ventilatory-response field test, popularly known as the "Can You Speak Comfortably?" threshold field test, compared to sophisticated laboratory tests that measure the same thing? "It is within spitting distance of the results from the laboratory tests," Carl says, explaining that it's close enough to lab accuracy that 90 percent of people are going to find it very useful to test and later retest to measure this key biomarker, T_1, and its higher-threshold sibling, T_2. Now, although I am a big proponent of VO_2 lab testing for accuracy in threshold detection and changes, the convenience and ease of an on-the-spot T_1 test can't be beat. It almost seems too easy: Just recite the "Pledge of Allegiance" (or something of a similar length that you know by heart).

Of course, before you say it, warm up a bit, and then run for two or three minutes at the slowest pace you can and measure that pace. Near the end of that two- or three-minute period (either on a treadmill or after taking a lap around a standard track), recite the "Pledge of Allegiance" out loud and ask yourself, "Can I speak comfortably?"

If the answer is yes, speed up (0.5 mph [1 kmph] on the treadmill is a good increment) and repeat the process. Eventually, you will find yourself equivocating, saying something to the effect of "Yeah, I can talk comfortably, but . . . ." Here, you've reached the transition point at T_1.

If you are wearing your heart rate monitor, your heart rate at the last speed which you answered "yes" is your T_1 heart rate. If you were hooked up to a metabolic cart in the laboratory, the lab staff would be seeing you reach your ventilatory threshold. Later, if you try to run at this pace, it will be too fast, by just a little bit. But if you slow down, by 0.5 mph to 1 mph (1 kmph to 2 kmph), you will find yourself at a comfortable pace that you can sustain for quite a long time.

If you want the long version, follow these eleven steps:

1. Put on your heart rate monitor and turn off the monitor's zone alarms (audible or visual).

2. Go to a track or a treadmill and begin with an adequate warm-up for five minutes.

3. Each stage is two minutes long. Starting at a speed of 5 mph (8 kmph), or as slowly as you can run on the track, increase your effort or intensity by 0.5 mph (1 kmph), or the smallest speed increment that you can make for each two-minute stage. Time the lap duration or record the speed.

4. One and a half minutes into each exercise stage (or as you enter the home stretch on the track), recite the "Pledge of Allegiance" out loud. You can use any standard thirty- to fifty-word paragraph in place of the "Pledge of Allegiance" if you do not know it by heart.

5. After the recitation, ask this one question: "Can I speak comfortably?"

6. There are only three answers that you may select: yes (+), not sure or uncertain (+/−), or no (−).
   • **Yes (+):** This means unequivocally, without a doubt, you can speak comfortably.
   • **Not sure or uncertain (+/−):** This means maybe, possibly, doubtful. If you find yourself qualifying a "yes" answer in any way, you have arrive at the +/− point.
   • **No (−):** This means you cannot speak comfortably.

After each two-minute interval, enter a sign that matches your answer in the table that follows.

1. Continue to increase your effort steadily until you answer "not sure" or "uncertain" and write it down (+/−).

2. Look back at your previous response. The last "yes" or plus sign (+), called the "last positive," is your T_1 speed and your T_1 heart rate. Your highest sustainable pace is likely to be one stage before the last (+) positive stage. The associated heart rate (bpm) when you reached this level of intensity or effort with the (+/−) point is likely to be approximately 80 percent of your maximal heart rate and your RPE is likely to be approximately 5 (i.e., hard).

3. Use the Heart Zones Threshold Heart Rate chart to set your five training zones. Here's the form that Carl uses for this test:

SPEED	LAP TIME	HEART RATE	TALK TEST RESULT

This is a sample chart you can use to set your five training zones.

1. You now have a choice to stop the test or to continue. I recommend that you stop the test because what you need is your speed and heart rate number coupled to T_1. If you are fairly fit and would like an estimate of T_2, the second or high threshold, you can choose to continue the sequence until your answer to the question in step 5 is "no." This will give you a direct measurement of your speed and heart rate at T_2.

2. Continue with the test. Your first negative (–), when you say "no, I cannot speak comfortably," is your T_2, or high threshold. This heart rate intensity is approximately 90 percent of your maximum heart rate or an RPE of a 7 (i.e., very hard). At an RPE of 7, you cannot recite the "Pledge of the Allegiance" (or your recitation of choice) without difficulty or without breathing uncomfortably. That's why ratcheting up the test to T_2 is not for beginners, unfit persons, or those returning to fitness activities.

According to Carl, there are a few tricks to making the threshold field test more accurate:

- Do the test at least two different times to reduce error. It can be done on the same day. Take at least a ten- to twenty-minute break between the two tests.

- Do the test on an easy-to-control piece of cardio equipment such as a treadmill, or a cycle ergometer if you want to use cycling for training. But remember that the response is activity-specific, so your heart rate at T_1 while you are running may not be exactly the same as your heart rate at T_1 while you are cycling. You can control speed and gradient increases more precisely than walking/jogging/running outside, where you must estimate your effort levels rather than using electronic dashboard information. Remember that this is a speed- or power-output-based test. Your heart rate (just like your ability to talk) is a response to changes in speed and power output. This test doesn't work nearly as well if you just try to ramp up your heart rate.

- Enlist a Heart Zones CPT (Certified Personal Trainer) by visiting the Heart Zones USA website (www.heartzones.com). CPTs have experience with the assessment and know the protocol to facilitate the test in order to eliminate error.

- If you are a multisport athlete, take the test while performing each sport activity, because threshold heart rates are sport-specific.

- If you have a speed and distance monitor that can measure your running pace, use it. Find out your pace, or the minutes per mile (or kilometer) that you are running at your first and low thresholds.

Remember: T_1 is a crossover point. Below this point, you should be able to sustain exercise for a long time very comfortably, and should be able to talk comfortably during training. Above this point, your sustainable exercise time decreases noticeably, and speech during training will be strained. T_2 is also a crossover point. Above this point, your sustainable exercise time is markedly reduced (less than twenty minutes) and speech is limited to single words, at best.

Physiologically, T_1 is a crossover point in both ventilation and lactate accumulation. That means that up until that point, exercise intensity and ventilation both increase in a linear manner. Then, at crossover (T_1), the ventilatory demands become greater than your body's ability to meet the oxygen required. At this intensity level and heart rate, ventilation increases exponentially rather than linearly; it is known as first ventilatory threshold (VT_1). The crossover point heart rate is nearly identical to the first lactate threshold intensity level. The discontinuity of linearity in either blood lactate accumulation or ventilatory patterns during incremental exercise represents a convenient marker of exercise training intensity.

The second threshold, T_2, occurs deeper into Zone 5, which is segmented into three subzones: Zone 5a, Zone 5b, and Zone 5c. I call these three the "hard, high, hot zones," reserved for those who love higher intensity and the wonderful benefits that are derived from the time spent there. T_2 is officially located between Zone 5a and Zone 5b, which puts it at around heart rate numbers that are 105 percent of your threshold heart rate. That means there is about a 6–10-bpm gap between the first and second threshold paces or heart rates. Of course, this difference is highly variable and unique to each person, and in large part is based on each person's physiology.

Those two subzones—5a and 5b—represent two distinct bodily responses: lactate clearance (5a) and maximum VO_2 (5b). Keep in mind that the Can You Speak Comfortably Foster Field Test yields an estimate of T_1 and T_2 and is not as precise as a lab test. An accurate measurement requires a formal metabolic assessment test; competitive athletes should periodically be retested to measure their fitness changes with this test.

APPLYING THRESHOLD TO HEART ZONES RUNNING

Now that you have your T_1, you're ready to apply it to the five-zone Heart Zones running construct and figure out how to train on a daily basis for your desired results.

The first step is to understand the benefits of each zone. Here are thumbnail descriptions:

- **Zone 1:** This low-intensity comfort zone, typified by easy walking/running that barely causes you to break a sweat, burns a low number of calories but provides some health benefits: lowered cholesterol, reduced stress, and improved blood pressure. This is an excellent intensity for cross-training.

- **Zone 2:** This easy zone, typified by low-intensity efforts that cause you to lightly break a sweat and can be maintained for long periods of time. You warm up and cool down in this zone, and you do your recovery workouts in this zone. As with Zone 1, cross-training at this kind of intensity allows you to recover both metabolically and in your joints.

- **Zone 3:** This moderate-intensity zone provides aerobic improvement benefits that include increases in the number of mitochondria, cardiac muscle strengthening, increased capillary density and profusion, improved fat utilization, and greater calorie burning than the lower zones. This is probably the intensity to use as you try to increase the duration of your longest training sessions.

- **Zone 4:** This sub-T_1 zone burns a lot of calories and causes significant improvement in aerobic capacity or cardiovascular fitness. This is probably the place where the bulk of your volume training will take place.

- **Zone 5a:** This above-T_1 zone has been described by Dr. Stephen Seiler, a Norwegian colleague of Carl's, as the "Black Hole" of training. In 5a, you are going too hard to really increase your training duration, but you aren't going hard enough to really challenge the ability of your heart to improve its cardiac output. If there is a single zone to avoid, this is it.

- **Zone 5b:** This high-intensity zone is for those who want to increase their VO_2 max (maximum volume of oxygen or maximal aerobic capacity). Most can only run in this zone for two- to eight-minute intervals without being forced to slow down and recover from the intensity. The 5b zone is highly stressful yet very important if you want to achieve your highest level of performance, but remember that this is the zone where you are training to race; it's way beyond the fitness area. As you get more and more accomplished, much of your training should be focused on building up time in this zone, but only to 10 percent of your training at this intensity, with the remaining bulk of your training in Zones 1–4.

ZONES/INTENSITY		% OF THRESHOLD	CALORIES BURNED (PER MIN.)	BENEFITS	WORKOUT TYPES	LOAD	WELLNESS ZONES	RPE	TALK	DESCRIPTORS	LACTATE
HEART ZONES TRAINING							**THRESHOLD ZONES**		**INTENSITY MEASUREMENTS**		
5 5c NEURO-MUSCULAR ZONE	AEROBIC	△ 110%	N/A	NEURO-MUSCULAR SPEED / FASTEST	EXPLOSIVE SPRINTS	90	PERFORMANCE ZONES	10	UNABLE	MAX. EFFORT	N/A
5b MAX. VO₂ ZONE	AEROBIC	110% TO 105%	>30	IMPROVED MAX. VO₂ / GET FASTEST	SHORT INTERVALS, SPEED DRILLS	30		9–10	GASPS	VERY, VERY HARD	>8
HIGH THRESHOLD (T₂)											
5a LACTATE CLEARANCE ZONE	NON-	105% TO 100%	>15	IMPROVED LACTATE CLEARANCE / GET FASTER	HIGH INTENSITY, SHORT CLIMBS	10		7–8	DIFFICULT	VERY HARD	3–8
LOW THRESHOLD (T₁)											
4 EXTREME AEROBIC ZONE	AEROBIC	100% TO 90%	~10	IMPROVED ENDURANCE / GET FITTER	INTERVALS *TWIST*	×4	FITNESS ZONES	5–6	HALTING	HARD	>2
3 HARD AEROBIC ZONE	AEROBIC	90% TO 80%	~7	IMPROVED ENDURANCE / GET FITTER	ENDURANCE STEADY-STATE	×3	ZONES	3–4	UNEASY	SOMEWHAT HARD	1–2
2 MODERATE AEROBIC ZONE	AEROBIC	80% TO 70%	~4	BUILD ENDURANCE / STAY FIT	LSD (LONG SLOW DISTANCE) RECOVERY	×2	HEALTH	2–3	NOT HARD	EASY	1
1 EASY AEROBIC ZONE	AEROBIC	70% TO 60%	~2	HEALTH BENEFITS / GET FIT	WARM UP COOL DOWN	×1		1–2	NO EFFORT	VERY EASY	<1

Figure 2.1

- **Zone 5c:** This all-out sprint zone is an above-the-stratosphere training intensity targeted mostly at improving muscle power, and should be reserved for the extremely fit. If you are merely looking for fitness, you do not need to spend any time in this zone.

Refer now to the accompanying Threshold Zones Chart **(see Figure 2.1)**. Read horizontally across the headings on the top row that give you details by zone of each of the following: zone number, intensity of threshold, benefits, workout types, load, wellness zones, and intensity measurements. This chart is the very core of the Heart Zones Threshold Training system because it provides you with the information you need to support training in different intensities and zones, to get different results.

HOW MUCH ARE YOU REALLY RUNNING? HERE'S A SIMPLE WAY TO MEASURE

The threshold running system is really powerful because it adds something that no other running program incorporates: how much and how hard you are running.

At its most basic level, the system allows you to measure how much you worked out. For example, if you want to train less but get the same effect that you got before you trained less, you need to push your workouts into a higher zone. After all, you can spend a lot of time in Zones 1 and 2 and not burn as many calories or get as much of a training effect (i.e., positive changes from the effort), or you can pick up the pace and move your effort into Zone 3 or 4 and get a whole lot of aerobic benefit and train for less time. What you just did in this instance is increase the training load.

Training load is the sum of all the stress that you put on your body: hills, road surfaces, weather, speed, time, and distance. It may help to think of load as analogous to weight. If you have a day of high volume and intensity, you've borne a heavy weight—a high load factor. Your load factor helps you gauge not only how much work you did, but also how much recovery you will need. A high-load day will require significant recovery time, whereas an easy day, with low distance and low zones, will allow you to go hard the next day. In this context, it is crucial that you get into the mindset that recovery days are not wasted training, but days where you prepare yourself to do the hard training that will lead to improvement. Good scientific data is emerging that demonstrates that the more you adopt a hard-day/easy-day approach, the more effective your training will be. In the words of Carl's Norwegian colleague and Stephen Seiler, Ph.D., "If you don't train easily enough to really recover on the easy days, you won't be able to train hard enough to improve on the hard days."

Along with the various kinds of training loads that runners can put on themselves, there are some unexpected loads you need to know about. One of these is emotional load—the weight from having an emotionally stressful day. Let's say your mom just got sick or the stock market dropped or you got in a huge argument with someone; each causes a lot of emotional weight. You know what it feels like when you can't run well because you just don't have the energy? That may well be caused by the stress from an emotionally difficult period. It is important to remember that hard training days and high unexpected loads don't mix. If you try to train hard when you aren't rested, or when you are emotionally upset, your body will rebel, usually by making you sick.

Another major load that runners experience is metabolic load. Metabolism is the sum of all of your energy input and output. Energy input is what you eat; if you eat well, eat healthy, and eat for your metabolism, your metabolic load is low. What happens when you eat junk or foods that you know are hard on your physiology? Yep, you raise your metabolic load. The same can be said for times when you are trying to lose weight by watching your diet particularly carefully. This is not a time to do your most intense training.

Quantifying every type of load that can tell you how much training you are doing is difficult to do. Too many factors are involved. Together, Carl and I have developed a point system which we call Heart Zones Training Points, or HZT Points. Carl has tested it in his lab to demonstrate that it works to quantify running load.

Best of all, it's a lot easier than counting calories. It'll give you data, numbers that take your running program to the next level, because it allows you to do the following:

- Compare your running workouts with each other.
- Compare one run with other runs.
- Compare your runs with those of other runners.
- Compare your runs with cross-training.

It's also important to see whether your running plan and the runs you actually did match each other—a huge factor. Carl has shown that one of the big causes of maladaptations to training comes from poor matching between the planned program and the executed program. We also want to acknowledge the contribution of Dr. Phil Skiba, who made very useful recommendations about how to modify the high end of the scale.

Here's how you calculate training load into HZT Points using our patented formula, called the LIFT equation:

- L = Load
- I = Intensity (weight for that zone number)
- F = Frequency (number of workouts)
- T = Time (minutes in each zone)
- where $L = I \times F \times T$, which equals running load.

ZONES	HZT POINTS PER MINUTE	HZT POINTS EARNED IN 10 MINUTES
Zone 1	1	10 points
Zone 2	2	20 points
Zone 3	3	30 points
Zone 4	4	40 points
Zone 5a	10	100 points
Zone 5b	30	300 points
Zone 5c	90	900 points

It's simple math that anyone can do. The above chart shows values that would be associated with ten minutes of exercise in each zone. If you stay in each zone for a continuous ten minutes, you will earn these points. However, it is important to note that the time in each zone is cumulative; it doesn't all have to be at the same time.

Now let's apply this to a real, thirty-minute, aerobic zones run:

- **5 minutes in Zone 2 = 5 × 2 = 10 points**
- **20 minutes in Zone 3 = 20 × 3 = 60 points**
- **5 minutes in Zone 4 = 5 × 4 = 20 points**

When you add up the running points, you get your total load—an HZT Points number—for your running workout. You can compare that day's HZT Points number to those of other days' workouts.

Given that one minute in Zone 2 gives you 2 points, one minute in Zone 3 is worth 3 points, and one minute in Zone 4 is worth four points, the preceding thirty-minute workout would earn you 90 points (10 + 60 + 20).

Over time, as you get fitter, you'll do more points per workout and per week. As you get fit enough, you'll regularly push past T_1 and into the red zone, Zone 5, where the load shifts from linear to exponential, provoking substantial gains in your fitness and giving you an exponential number of run-training points. However, you need to keep in mind that the time in Zones 5b and 5c should probably not be greater than 10 percent of your total training, and that the bulk of your training (70 percent to 80 percent) should be in Zones 1–4.

This way of measuring how much running stress you are experiencing is easier than counting calories. It's a way to prescribe running using a methodology that measures how much exercise you are getting. It's the only way to simply and quickly quantify cardiovascular training in a way that you can use for comparison and analysis over any time period.

Just remember the formula: time in the zone multiplied by the stress number assigned to that zone. It's easy. So, grab your heart rate monitor, because heart rate is what we'll calculate next.

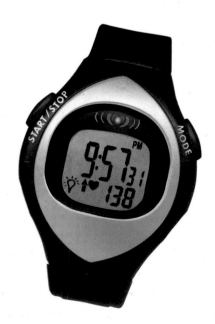

The Blink Heart Rate Monitor

ESTABLISHING YOUR OWN THRESHOLD ZONES

You've done the threshold talk test and found out where you no longer can speak comfortably, and you've found your first threshold, your T_1 heart rate. You know from that field test that T_1 is your 100 percent; it is, in relative measurements, your 100 percent anchor point. From that baseline, we will calculate the ceiling and floors, your zone limits, which in the threshold system look like this:

- Zone 1 is 60 percent to 70 percent of threshold heart rate
- Zone 2 is 70 percent to 80 percent of threshold heart rate
- Zone 3 is 80 percent to 90 percent of threshold heart rate
- Zone 4 is 90 percent to 100 percent of threshold heart rate

Low threshold:

- Zone 5a is 100 percent to 105 percent of threshold heart rate

High threshold:

- Zone 5b is 105 percent to 110 percent of threshold heart rate
- Zone 5c is greater than 110 percent of threshold heart rate

Now, do the math. If your threshold heart rate is 120 bpm, your Zone 4 heart rate range is 108 to 120 bpm. If your threshold heart rate is 180 bpm, your Zone 4 range is 162 to 180 bpm. Use the Threshold Heart Rate chart for zone limits ranging from 120 to 200 bpm.

The Heart Zones Training threshold sets up a logical framework for you and your heart rate monitor. You say, "Today I did a recovery workout (thirty minutes in Zone 2 = 60 HZT Points); tomorrow I want to do a very long workout (thirty minutes in Zone 3, ninety minutes in Zone 4 = 450 HZT Points). The next day I want to do another recovery workout (60 HRT Points). The day after that I

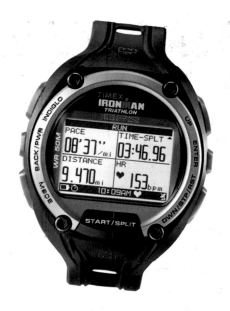

Timex Ironman Global Trainer

want to do a high-intensity workout (thirty minutes in Zone 3, ten minutes in Zone 5a, twenty minutes in Zone 5b = 790 HZT Points)."

If you do an hour of running, which is what I recommend people gradually work up to, you do a lot of Zone 3 and Zone 4 time, which are your best aerobic zones, because they are at a high enough intensity to stimulate a cardiovascular improvement in oxygen consumption, and you burn a high enough number of total calories. Walking doesn't really do it as well—it's too low-intensity to improve, but it's perfect for recovery training.

There are a lot of different ways to use training tools to make your run workouts easier and more powerful such as measuring the following: RPE, maximum heart rate, power watts, speed, and distance. The list goes on. But I know that threshold training works best. It is dynamic. It demands that you test and retest to see your fitness changes. It is motivational because it shows the improvements in your fitness. It is a simple way to train, and it gets results. How could you ask for more?

PROGRESSIVE CROSS-VARIABILITY TRAINING: A VARYING PLAN THAT UTILIZES CROSS-TRAINING AND PROGRESSES IN INTENSITY

I know that a lot of coaches take a lot of pride in devising varied, complex training strategies that are supposedly tailored specifically to the individual. Well, this plan, which we call Progressive Cross-Variability Training, is way different. It is the result of years of hunting for universal, scientifically rooted laws that apply to virtually everyone. It started with studies that analyzed the way real runners run, altered their training stimulus, combined it with the proven benefits of periodization and cross-training, and came up with these five very definite, logical guidelines for building better performance:

1. Run very, very hard in about 10 percent of your total workout time—but no more than that. That means at least once a week do a workout with intervals, which are efforts that range from thirty-second all-out bursts to somewhat faster-than-race-pace effort in the zone above T_2. Extra-long runs at a moderate pace also qualify as hard runs, although the 10 percent rule applies to high intensity only. These extraordinary efforts make you a stronger runner. They hyperstress your physiology and tear your body down, and then, when followed by a day or two of rest, build it up better than it was before.

2. Always follow a hard day with an easy day. Exercising for a short duration at a low-stress, low-zone, low-duration pace that allows you to conduct easy conversation gives your interval-battered muscles time to heal and improve. This day should be devoted to recovery, to preparing yourself for your next hard workout.

3. Spend as little time as possible in the "Between," moderately hard zone, the Black Hole. Beware of training in the moderately hard workout zone in which it is difficult to speak comfortably; this pace is not beneficial because it's both too easy and too hard: too easy to improve your VO_2 max, and too hard to allow recovery from a true hard day and allow you to go long enough to really work on endurance. If you run the same route and the same pace every day in this "Between" zone where you feel somewhat uncomfortable, but aren't really pushing super hard, you are putting yourself in a constant state of fatigue. That's why this zone, which is just above threshold (T_1) in the Heart Zones system, is called the Black Hole. Don't go there.

4. Cross-train—rarely run two days in a row. The best practice is to follow a running day with a cross-training day. Bike, swim, paddle, use an elliptical, row—do anything that will allow recovery from your run—or don't work out at all. Don't do hard cross-training workouts, as they are designed for recovery; even if cross-training works different muscles, the hard work won't let your overall metabolic system rest and recover. No matter what you do the day after a hard workout, take it easy.

5. In the weeks and months leading up to your race, progressively increase the training load on your hard days. Make your hard days harder and harder as you get fitter. This ramps you up to the peak fitness you'll need to do your best in an event.

BE LIKE BONNIE: WORK HARD AND HONOR THE RECOVERY DAY

Follow these five rules and you will get faster and greatly reduce your chances of injury. Here's the story of how we came up with them.

When Eric Heiden stunned the speedskating world by winning all five possible Olympic skating gold medals at the 1980 Olympic Games in Lake Placid, New York, an unprecedented and probably unrepeatable feat that included both short- and long-distance events, there was a hidden aftereffect: He made life hell for the athletes who followed him.

"His coaches thought 'great, we'll train everyone just like Eric trained,'" says Carl Foster. "After all, coaches are famous for copying the training of their last champion. With Heiden, they thought they'd found the right formula. The trouble was that his physiology was unique—he could train hard every day. The average guy—even the average world-class athlete—just can't handle that kind of workload for very long."

Nearly every human—except for the truly marvelous exceptions like Heiden (who also went on to a second career as a Tour de France cyclist)—requires at least forty-eight hours (not a mere twenty-four) to recover from a hard workout. "Without following a hard day with an easy day, most athletes will destroy themselves in training," says Foster. He finds that athletes are notorious for overworking on the day the coach scheduled recovery training, spoiling even the best-designed programs.

Four-time Olympian Bonnie Blair, who won five speed-skating gold medals and a bronze in a spectacular career that spanned Olympic Games from 1984 to 1994, seemed to instinctively know about the need for recovery. That's why, struggling a bit during a period leading up to the 1992 Olympics, she changed coaches and stopped talking to Foster for nearly two years.

"She had remarkable technique, and is the most competitive soul and 'Eye of the Tiger' personality that I've ever seen. But she had a fairly normal physiology for a world-class athlete," explains Foster. "So, she needed more rest than the coaches were giving her." Within months, Bonnie got her winning groove back—all because she refused to be trained like Heiden.

Whenever Foster crossed paths with her during that period, Blair ignored him. "Why were you pissed at me?" he asked a few years later. "She said, 'Well, your job was to tell the coaches to let us take a day off. And if you didn't, what good are you as a physiologist?'" Carl was speechless. She was right.

"I had actually looked at test results too coldly, without looking at the skaters' faces," Carl says. "They had come back from an early season camp in Europe looking very tired, but I looked only at the blood lactate and the VO_2 results and, quite honestly, forgot that looking into the athletes' eyes is the most important test one does."

The lesson here? Since the vast majority of people, even very good athletes, are born with physiologies more like Bonnie's than Eric's, you absolutely need rest/recovery days. If you want to get stronger and faster, and you are not a totally unique, once-in-a-lifetime athlete like Heiden, just remember four words: Go hard/go easy. Follow a very hard day by a very easy day. In fact, you should usually follow a very hard day with two easy days.

HOW HARD IS HARD?

In Heart Zones Training (HZT) parlance, the hard days accumulate lots of training points. They either take you to the "Above" zones, above T_2—the high-intensity Zones 5b and 5c, 105 percent to 110 percent, and 110+ percent of threshold heart rate—or they build up duration in Zone 4. Also, although we will normally speak of "hard" in terms of training intensity, in HZT language the real test of whether a day was hard or easy is how you describe your training day when you lay your head on the pillow in the evening. Whether it is three hours in Zone 4 or thirty minutes in Zone 5b, when you lie down in the evening you are going to know it was "hard."

Conversely, how easy is easy? Go back to the ACSM recommendation for moderate exercise. In Heart Zones Training parlance, the easy days never take you above T_1; you're in HZT Zones 2–4 which is 70 percent to 99 percent of your threshold heart rate. You are in the "Below" zones.

Because everything has to have a name, I call this variability training (the "progressive" and the "cross-" will come soon), because you must vary your workouts to get a training effect. Use hard days to push your body to get better. Follow those with easy days to rest, recover, and let your body strengthen.

Hard days put a high load on your body they are designed to be stressful enough that the body tells itself to adapt by getting stronger and faster. But it is on the easy days, the short-duration, low-stress workout days, when recovery from the hard workout takes place, and the body actually rebuilds itself stronger.

If you run every day at high speed or high intensity, or even for a longer time than usual at a low intensity, you may overload your body with stress to the point where you do more harm (negative adaptation), rather than gaining positive adaptation. That's why a hard day must be followed by an easy day.

Don't get lazy. "For best results, make the hard days very, very hard and the easy days very easy, and don't ever do two hard days in a row," says Carl. "Unless you are among the one out of a million people like Eric Heiden who can train with minimal rest (and remember that Eric thought he was doing easy, recovery training; but for everyone else it was still pretty hard), you must build in recovery time. That's when your body actually heals up and gets stronger." Whatever you do, try to avoid the Black Hole.

BEWARE THE BLACK HOLE AND MONOTONY TRAINING

The Black Hole, a key concept in this book, is the name that, exercise physiologist Dr. Stephen Seiler of Agdar University, gave to a detrimental pace that most runners run in too much of the time.

"The Black Hole is running at an effort that feels a little hard but not at a real hard training intensity," says Carl. "It's that in-between, can't-really-talk-too-well place where you are not training at a high enough intensity to improve VO_2 max but not long enough to really build endurance, and certainly not easy enough to recover."

Staying in the Black Hole for thirty or forty-five minutes day after day—which many people do, running their same route over and over—results in a lack of variation in training load that Carl calls "training monotony," a recipe

for stagnation and injury. But also keep in mind that you can even get training monotony if the training is varied, but always hard, as are a short interval session and a long run. "When your training monotony is high, it makes you too tired to run hard on the hard days," says Carl. "Add frequent injuries, and you just don't improve."

Your body needs day-to-day variation—high-intensity training or high volume with low-intensity training followed by a regular cycle of rest and recovery, within the week as well as between weeks. When you don't get this variation, often you will take an involuntary rest, by catching a cold or injuring yourself.

Technically, the Black Hole is a suboptimal training zone that is roughly between a marathon and 10K pace. It's a surprisingly narrow space. In the Heart Zones Training System, it would be an intensity level between T_1 and T_2, which translates to Zone 5a, or approximately 100 percent to 105 percent of your threshold heart rate.

Black Hole identifier Stephen Seiler, who recognized the problem of this less-effective training intensity and applied the astronomical term to it, was among the first to conduct studies that examined the training distribution of serious athletes. His idea was that well-trained athletes around the world would, through a Darwinian process of trial-and-error and word of mouth, end up doing the most efficient training. At the kind of training loads undertaken by elite athletes, training mistakes are very unforgiving.

Seiler found that serious endurance athletes (runners, skiers, cyclists, rowers) only spend about 10 percent over T_2 (interval-style high-intensity training, or Zones 5b and 5c) and 70 percent to 80 percent of their training time at a pace lower than T_1 (Zones 1–4). It seems that they only spend about 10 percent to 20 percent of their time in the Black Hole. Then he and Carl joined a study led by a Spanish colleague, Dr. Jonathan Esteve-Lanao of the European University of Madrid, which tested whether spending more or less time in the Black Hole would have an effect on performance.

Esteve-Lanao (who is a coach in addition to being a Ph.D. physiologist) first tested a group of Spanish runners and reported similar training percentages as Seiler's when he let the runners train using his normal training plan. Then, fixing 8 percent of their training in high-intensity intervals (he had later concluded that around 10 percent interval training was all runners' bodies could handle), he divided his test subjects into two groups and modified the amount of training time each spent in the other two zones, the Black Hole and an easy, sub-T_1 pace. One group did 80/12/8: 80 percent in the easy zone, 12 percent in the Black Hole, and 8 percent at the hard T_2 + interval pace. The other group trained in a 67/25/8 ratio.

Then, after five months, they raced the same distance they had at the start of the study: 6.5 miles (10.4 km). The result: Both groups had improved, but the group that did less time in the Black Hole improved 26 percent more: 157 seconds versus 121 seconds.

Now, it might seem counterintuitive that the group that took it easier in training would run faster on race day—and the researchers can't give a definitive explanation why. But Carl guesses that the answer simply is better recovery. After all, the 12 percent Black Hole group had much more recovery time in the sub-T_1 pace zone (80 percent) than did the 25 percent Black Hole group (67 percent).

Would zero Black Hole training time result in faster speeds? That hasn't been researched yet, but it makes sense. "Your body responds better to the harder training (greater than T_2) when it is more rested," says Carl. He notes, however, that some time in the Black Hole—say, 10 percent to 20 percent of your training—is probably unavoidable, as you would pass through this intensity on the way up and the way down during high-intensity training days.

Carl also speculates that training in the Black Hole desensitizes your body to adrenaline, the hormone that lets you really get excited for races. He can't back this desensitization theory with any hard data, but he does offer an analogy to how it might work: your sense of smell.

When you enter a room with a pungent odor (say, a gas station rest room) it will be repulsive at first. But stay in that room long enough, and soon it doesn't bother you as much, as if your nose doesn't work as well. And it doesn't—it has been desensitized.

Even though the Black Hole is a relatively small sliver of your heart rate spectrum—about 100 percent to 105 percent of threshold—earnest, hard-working runners camp out way too much there. Sometimes it's the only pace runners train at or know. That's because it's a very attractive place: just hard enough to make us feel that we're doing some good. Add the addictive runner's-high effect, and you don't want to leave the Hole. But if you want to get faster, you have to snap out of the endorphin trance and recognize that the Black Hole is like training purgatory.

So, the rule is clear: If you want to improve, avoid injuries, and stay excited about your sport, vary your workouts. Go really hard on hard days and go really short and easy on easy days. And keep out of the Black Hole.

MARRYING PERIODIZATION AND CROSS-TRAINING

To get a lot fitter, to do your best in your chosen race, whether it is the Olympics or the World Championships or your local 5K, you must apply the hard/easy scenario progressively. That means over the weeks and months of building up to the big day, the hard days must get even harder and/or longer than the previous hard days—all while the easy days stay sacrosanct. In fact, to make sure your body does not reach race day overstressed and overtrained, you must schedule an easy week every month to consolidate the gains.

If this mix-and-match system of hard-and-easy work days and weeks that progressively get harder up to peak fitness sounds vaguely familiar to you, give yourself a pat on the back. It's been used in some form by runners, weight lifters, and all endurance athletes for decades. It's called periodization.

The foundation of all modern training, periodization was developed in the early 1960s by Romania's Tudor Bompa, a coach and former Olympic rower who built his athletes up to top game-day form with a stairstep series of methodical, progressive challenges and recoveries. It breaks your training into four ascending periods (training phases) that vary the volume, timing, and intensity of workouts. This "planned variation," as many call it, stops your fitness from reaching a plateau (as it does when you run the same miles or kilometers at the same pace every day) by delivering a continual combination of stress and rest along a trend line of increased volume that keeps your aerobic and structural systems simultaneously improving. Periodization brings you to peak form with a penultimate phase of speedwork and reduced volume, and then adds a taper to leave you fresh for race day.

There is really no arguing against periodization; it is so well proven at this point that it is practically the athletic-training gospel. It's the antithesis of old-fashioned monotony training that leaves everyone so stale. But periodization is not the last word; I think it can be improved immeasurably by stirring in a missing ingredient: cross-training.

A LOOK AT WHAT CROSS-TRAINING CAN DO

My emphasis on cross-training surely will not come as a surprise to anyone who knows of my history in triathlons. But don't simply write that off as my personal obsession. Some single-sport athletes had been tapping cross-training power long before triathlons came along, but nobody knew it. It isn't mere coincidence that we started off this chapter with speedskaters, because they are among the world's most dedicated cross-trainers. They use running, riding, swimming, weight training, and more to train for speed-skating on ice, because until very recently there were no indoor speedskating rinks.

And just as cross-training works for skaters, I believe it can work for runners, particularly in the early months of periodization, when you are building your base. In fact, I know it can, because swimming and cycling unwittingly helped me set my marathon PR. Here's the story:

In 1972 at age twenty-five, just back from a year of working as a Red Cross volunteer in Vietnam, I starting running seriously, doing the Bay to Breakers and other "fun runs," as we called them back then. By the late 1970s and early 1980s, that led to ultra-marathons and Ironman triathlons, and my running grew to 100-mile (161 km) weeks.

The whole time I was totally self-coached. There were no running programs for women in college; there was no *Title 9*, which funds programs for women. I started experimenting. From the world of track and field, there was interval training—high intensity/low volume. I started drawing my training plan from the writings of people like Joe Henderson, the editor of *Runners' World*, and Arthur Lydiard, the famous New Zealand icon who developed LSD—long, slow distance, progressively adding volume.

Anyhow, I started turning myself into a little lab rat. I practiced LSD for eight weeks. Hmmm . . . that didn't go very well. So, I added intervals and whatever else I'd heard about. Soon, I was combining them all in one week: one day of hills, for strength; two days of speed training, one at the track and the other on the road; low-zone volume training—classic LSD; and then a once-a-week time trial.

Even before I started cross-training, I liked this vari-ability training. It was making me feel incredibly fit. And it was working.

After running my first marathon in 1976 (the Silver State Marathon near Reno, Nevada), I won the Sacramento (California) Marathon in 1977 and 1978. I set the Oklahoma state marathon record in 1979, and won the Tortuous 26 marathon in the depth of Minnesota winter in January. It was so cold that morning that all the aid stations had to heat the water so that it wouldn't freeze on our lips.

I found that the longer and longer I went, the more I won. So, I kept the variability, kept out of the Black Hole that Carl and the other physiologists would discover twen-ty years later, and stayed on my quest to answer the ques-tion "How far and how fast can the human body run?"

Then I added cross-training—and had the best running performances of my life, winning the Western States 100 in 1980 and qualifying for the 1984 Olympic trial with my marathon PR. Doing so convinced me that cross-training can help any runner, from recreational runner to hard-bitten racer, run better at any distance.

Yes, I realize that statement may fly in the face of run-ning purists who argue that sports specificity rules—that to get better at any sport, you have to train 100 percent of the time in that sport. Specificity does have its place as part of a training program. But for the majority of the time, cross-training is the best use of your training time.

I know it because it helped me become part of history—to run in the first U.S. Olympic trials to select the U.S. women for the first-ever women's Olympic marathon, to be held in the 1984 Games in Los Angeles. At the time, the longest women's race in the Games had been a measly 5K.

The Olympic Organizing Committee said that they'd pay the travel expenses for the top 200 women marathon-ers in the country to meet at the starting line in Olympia, Washington, to select the first women's U.S. marathon team, but there was one caveat: You had to have previously run a 2:51 marathon to make the cut.

Yikes! My marathon PR at the time was a so-so 2:55. I excelled at longer races, such as the Western States 100 and the prestigious American River 50 Miler, which I won in 1979.

On top of that, I was thirty-seven years old in 1983, not exactly in my prime anymore. Moreover, I wasn't even a pure runner by then, having jumped whole hog into triathlon. In fact, after doing my first triathlon in 1978, I had morphed into a bona fide multisport star, taking second place at the Hawaii Ironman in 1981 and third twice in 1982 (the race was held in both February and its new October date that year). I was a top-rated threat for 1983.

Bottom line: I was an experienced but borderline national-class marathoner required to cut my PR marathon time by four minutes—about nine seconds per mile—while on the downside of my running career as I trained for another sport. To the logical mind, it probably didn't sound like a good bet. But, of course, I had a plan—a plan that was literally forced on me.

To bag the 2:51 qualifying time that it would take to get me into the Olympic trials, I targeted the Phoenix (Arizona) Marathon in February 2004. It was a course well suited to a PR: flat, flat, flat with cool winter desert temperatures. Race directors were advertising ideal weather conditions—a typical off-season Phoenix was ideal for me. Now, to build my base for that race, I had to do something that no running coach in his or her right mind would recommend: cross-train. Actually, I couldn't do anything about that—I was a sponsored triathlete. So, I would simply do my normal Ironman training through October 2003, go to Kona and race the Ironman, and then switch to all running for fourteen weeks. Simple, right?

So, I swam-biked-ran all summer. I did the 1983 Ironman, taking fifth place. Then I did R&R (rest and recovery) training for four weeks. Starting November 1, I didn't touch my goggles or my bike; I trained only in running shoes over the next fourteen weeks, rebuilding my running base with LSD for two weeks, building strength by progressively adding hills over the next two weeks, adding speed for the next two weeks, and then mixing it up. Each day had a purpose. It led me to the discovery of a model that I coined "the Training Tree": Every two weeks I'd climb up a branch to more training load and harder workouts. By the end of eight weeks, I'd be ready. I then tapered and flew to Phoenix for the moment of truth.

I ran a 2:50:15 marathon, my PR. I was going to Olympia, baby! I was one of the 200 fastest women in the United States, and I had a chance to make history.

It didn't matter three months later that I finished in the middle of the pack with a 3:05, running stride for stride with one of my heroes, the amazing Sister Marion Irvine, a fifty-one-year-old Catholic girls school principal and the oldest woman ever to qualify for an Olympic trials event. The lesson I came away with from this experience was a valuable one that I had theorized about for years, and now was sure could benefit every runner: Cross-training makes runners better at running.

THE SCIENCE BACKS IT UP

My experience jives with research from Carl, who found that cross-training was great for overall fitness and base building, and offers long-term health and anti-injury and performance benefits, but that pure, sports-specific running training was faster in the short term.

In 1995, Carl did a study of casual "t-shirt runners," as he calls them, whom he split into three groups:

- **Group 1:** controls who maintained easy training
- **Group 2:** a periodized group that observed a hard/easy training format and added more running
- **Group 3:** a periodized group that added swimming to the baseline level of running

By the end of the training test period, Group 1 had no speed gains in a 2-mile (3 km) run, Group 2 (the pure runners) cut thirty seconds off their 2-mile time, and Group 3 cut fifteen seconds off.

"To get serious about running fast, ultimately you have to run," says Carl. "But the cross-training can work for base building and your recovery days."

As I've aged, I've come to see cross-training as a critical link in all levels of running.

The variety of available cross-training options is such that even the most hard-bitten runner will find some kind of nonrunning cardio to like: swimming, bicycling, elliptical machine, aerobics, even ballroom dancing. Nowadays, in addition to biking and swimming, I row and in-line skate. In the winter I snowshoe, sled (yes, interval training with runs up the hills dragging my sled), snowboard, and cross-country ski. A few years from now, I might be doing something different as new sports and new interests arise. And that will be great, because cross-training makes you, as I like to say, "365-Fit"—so all-around fit that your body is able to handle virtually any crazy thing that comes along for a significant period of time. 365-Fit means being able to do anything at any time. If a biker buddy of mine calls up and says "let's ride a century," I can do that with no preparation. If the task is to climb a 14,000-foot (4,267 m) mountain, I can do that. If a pal wants to hike the Machu Picchu trail in Peru, I can do that (in fact, I did that). If there is a challenge in some far-out thing I've never done—Colorado river boarding, Bolivian mine shaft climbing Greenlandic ice-cap glassading, you name it—I can and will do it. Believe me, you never get bored cross-training and living the lifestyle of 365-Fit.

One warning about cross-training, however: Don't go too hard. You might think that you could follow a hard running day with a hard swim, given the upper-body focus of the latter. But Carl warns that doing that will hurt you by allowing only partial recovery.

"The orthopedic part—your muscles and connective tissue—can recover with cross-training because activities like cycling, swimming, and elliptical unload your muscles and skeleton," he says. "But the metabolic part (heart, lungs, respiratory and circulatory systems) don't know the difference—and can't recover. To them, work is work. So, if you follow a hard run with a hard swim, bike, or paddle, you'll still be tired from the day before."

The bottom line is that cross-training will benefit you in and out of your running shoes. It can and should be used during all phases of running by all runners—competitive and recreational alike.

The key: You must find the types of cross-training that work for you, that you enjoy doing. Then you must be sure to do it—and do it in the right way, that is, in a manner that enhances and does not disrupt your running program.

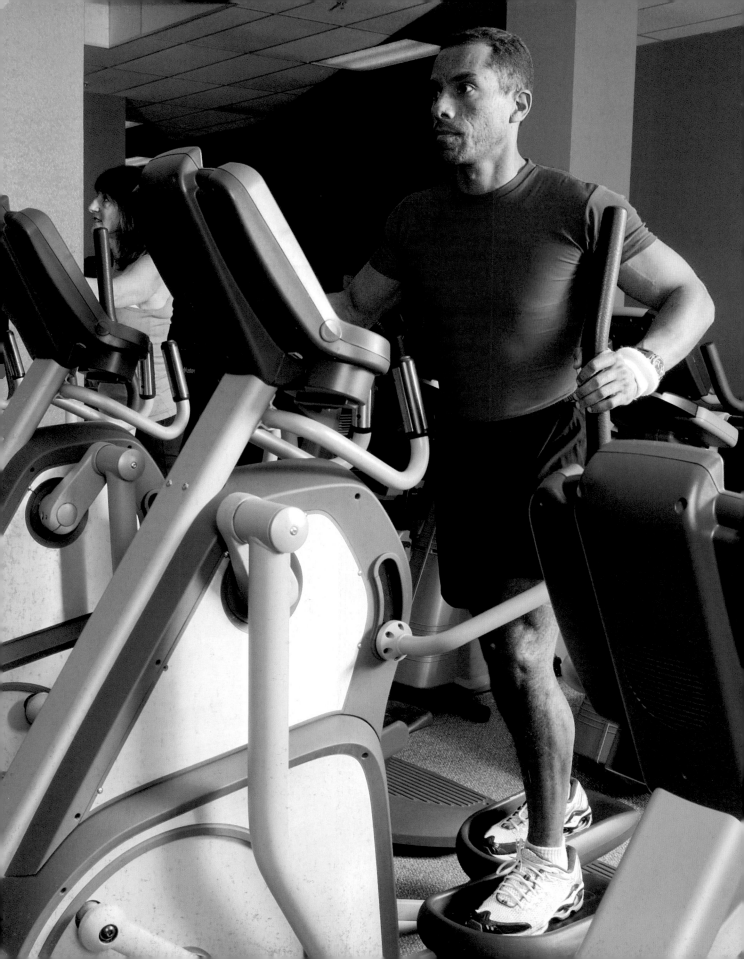

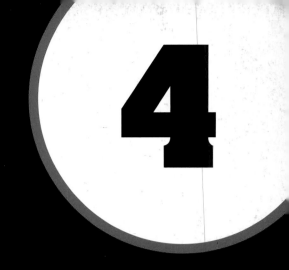

STRENGTH TRAINING AND CROSS-TRAINING: BUILDING ALL-BODY FITNESS

MANY RUNNERS HAVE A PROBLEM: They still have the same attitude that they had in the 70s or the 80s or even the 90s: running just involves running.

Well, we're smarter than that today. Research in the past few decades and simple common sense tell us now that running is not enough, that doing the same left-right, left-right over and over without mixing in other activities leaves your mind bored and your body more susceptible to repetitive-motion injuries. We know that ceaseless aerobic activity, partnered with no specific strengthening exercises, tends to wear down muscle mass. We know that the lack of stretching and flexibility leads to imbalances that slow you down and lead to injuries. Mono-sport bodies break down more often than strong, balanced, and functionally resilient bodies. When we look at life in the long run, we know that multisport, strength-hardened, well-stretched bodies go faster, last longer, and get fewer injuries.

So, if these benefits are so well known, you might ask, why do we runners just keep running—and nothing else? Why do so few runners go to the gym, hit the weights, and stretch?

I don't know for sure; I'm not a psychologist. Maybe the sheer addictiveness of the endorphin-fueled runner's high compels runners to sweep aside common sense and good long-term fitness advice that will actually help their running. But as a runner who has spent a large chunk of my career involved in the sport of triathlon, I can tell you this: If you ignore the trio of strength training, cross-training, and stretching, you do it at your own peril.

CROSS-TRAINING ALTERNATIVES FOR RECOVERY AND REHAB

Daily running, whether it's long or short, high-intensity or low-intensity, is hard on everybody, young and old. Every run, just as with every weight training like session, causes some degree of damage (i.e., micro-tears) in muscle tissue. Those tears actually strengthen the muscle when given time, as they turn on the signal to make more and better muscle tissue. The trouble is that daily running does not allow that recovery time. Most people use a ballpark figure of at least forty-eight hours to recover from a weight session. So, the question is "How do I make time for recovery from a run or from a running-caused injury, but stay in running shape?"

The answer is to broaden your athletic portfolio. On your recovery days, mix in swimming, rowing, cycling, elliptical machine, aerobic dance, whatever. Use that VersaClimber machine at the gym that no one touches. Try a Trikke, the self-powered three-wheeled scooter that you power by torquing your body side to side. Because what I'm talking about here is my old multisport friend: cross-training.

The truth is that your VO_2 max isn't particular about what aerobic activity you choose to develop it. The central cardiovascular benefits from cross-training are still present, allowing your running muscles to work without losing the basis of your aerobic capacity. Cross-training helps you keep your hard workouts, and can't be beat for convenience. Two straight days of running is tough on your body, but one day of hard running followed by a swim session lets your legs recover while it works your upper body, with both blasting your heart and lungs.

Going on a business trip? Tuck swim goggles into your suitcase along with your running shoes. Really tweak your knee? Rent a kayak for a couple of days. Can't run due to a January blizzard and subzero temps? Snowshoe, cross-country ski, or hit the elliptical machine at the club. Mixing up different activities—including road running and trail running—keeps you motivated, breaks up your routine, and helps maintain fitness. Unless you are a high-level racer who must solely practice sport-specific training to be competitive, cross-training is the healthiest way to go. Other sports not only don't hurt your running training, but also can provide a variety that keeps you from getting bored with it. In some cases, cross-training can even provide strength training.

Cross-training shouldn't be seen simply as a welcome off-season break from a season of running races, and something to set aside when spring rolls around. Because it works all the muscles of the body rather than just a specific group, cross-training reduces the risk of chronic injury over the long term compared to any one sport. And in the big picture, cross-training makes you fitter, enhancing VO_2 max by developing oxygen-processing ability in all muscles of the body, not just the ones in your legs.

COMMON CROSS-TRAINING ALTERNATIVES

I cross-train all year because it allows my sport-specific muscles—my running muscles—to rest while I still train my other metabolic and physiological systems such as my heart and lungs, and my energy-burning capacity.

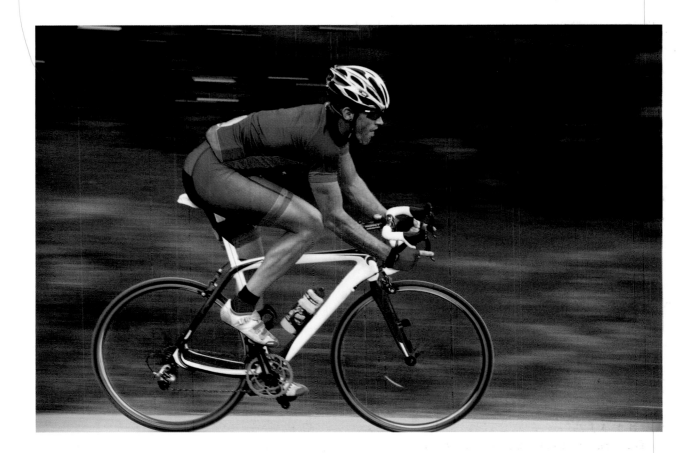

CYCLING

A leg-centric exercise like running, but so easy on the knees and effective at transporting nutrient-rich blood to leg muscles that it is often prescribed as therapy for rehabbing runners, cycling can have a unique healing effect on runners' legs the day after a hard run. That is because it does a great job of funneling huge quantities of blood nutrients to running muscles without the ballistic shock that causes injuries and large quantities of micro-tears. A five-minute spin on a stationary trainer is also very healing immediately after a run. How about performance? Can cycling help runners maintain their running fitness—or even improve it? The answer is possibly. There have been many studies and many results, ranging from a minor, sometimes inconsequential fall-off in fitness to some long-term improvement, factoring in reduced injuries from less running. My conclusion is that you can maintain running fitness by replacing some of your running with cycling—as long as the cycling includes a great deal of intensity. (At the same time, I believe that low-intensity cycling is the perfect way to manage your recovery days. It is low-intensity metabolically, giving your body the kind of deep recuperation time it needs from hard running workouts, plus it's not orthopedically challenging, so your feet, knees, and hips can recover.)

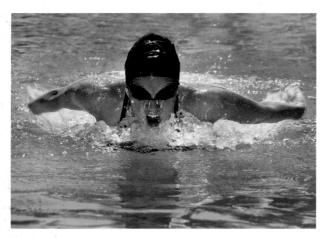

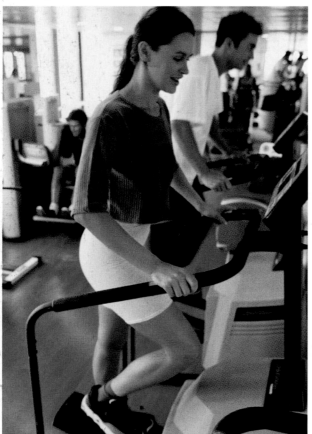

SWIMMING

An almost-perfect complement to running, this upper-body-centric activity gives your legs a rest, straightens your posture, works your core, hammers your heart, and gives you the superb upper-body development completely ignored by running. A study by Carl at the Milwaukee Heart Institute found that supplemental swimming improved runners' 2-mile (3 km) times by fifteen seconds. Although that was only half the thirty-second speed gains that runners who added more running training made, the researchers theorized that the risk of injuries would be reduced in the swimmers compared to the pure runners. Thus, if you are near your specific training limit, cross-training with swimming can add somewhat to your specific running ability.

HIKING/STAIRSTEPPING

This bipedal activity is quite different from running. It works a different set of muscles, and, for the most part, does not involve the pounding on the knees and feet that comes with running. A study cited by Brian Whitesides, MPT, on Betterrunner.com reported that the stairstepper machine was the only cross-training mode that improved running times without increasing overall workout times. In other words, although the swimming study cited in the preceding section added swimming on top of a preexisting running program, stairstepping can replace some running, therefore not adding to workout time. Note that this study was conducted on "fit" college students who were not run-specific athletes.

IN-LINE SKATING

Another bi-pedal alternative that works abductors and adductors in a different way than running is in-line skating. The forceful push to the outside is a superb way to build the glutes, often underutilized in running but essential for balance and injury reduction, particularly in reducing knee pain and IT band syndrome. Research conducted at the University of Wisconsin found that skating and treadmill running had similar heart rate and oxygen-use patterns. The big downside, however, is literally the down side: The risk of injuries from falling in in-line skating is significant.

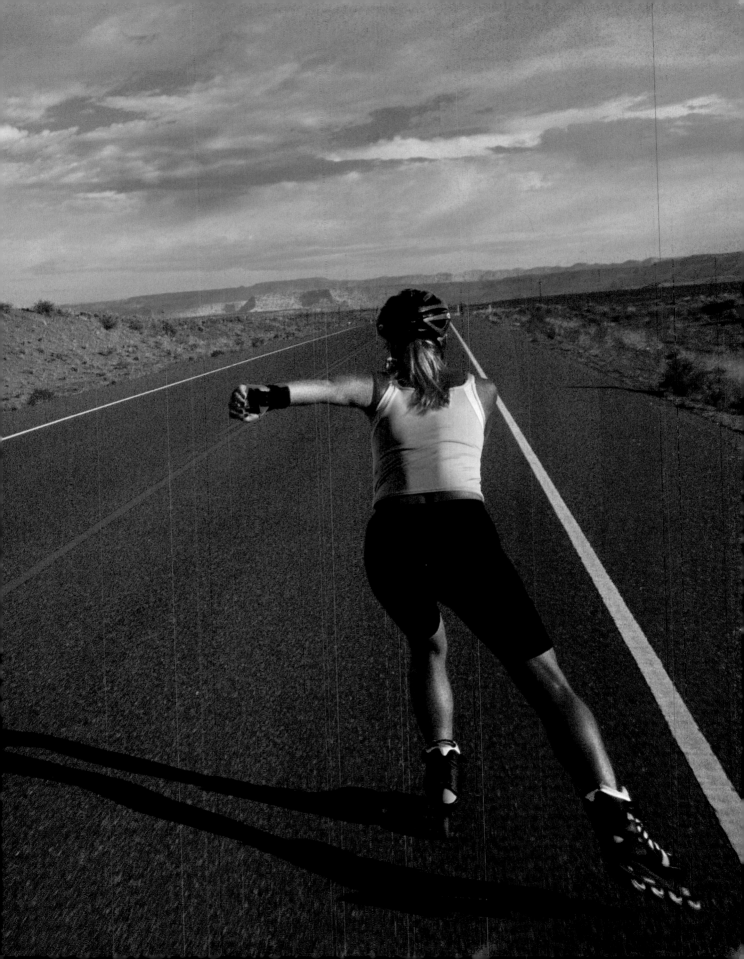

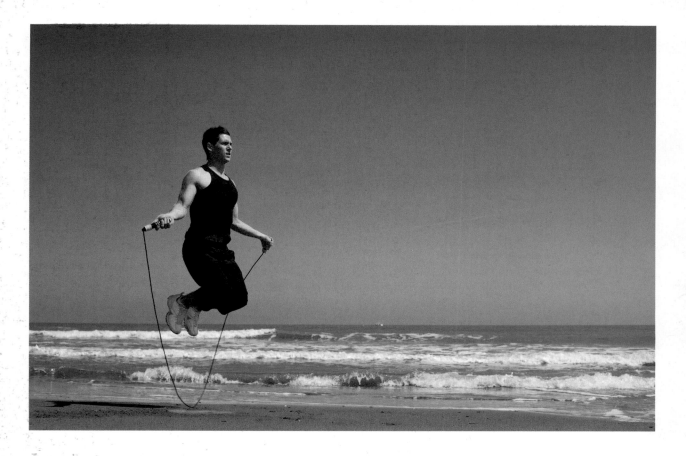

JUMPING ROPE

The single most convenient aerobic activity in the world because it can be done anywhere, jumping rope is an interesting, low-impact alternative that strengthens calves, builds coordination, and promotes general fitness. It is not as aerobic as some of the other cross-training options, but it can be quite a workout if you challenge yourself with different jumping styles.

ELLIPTICAL MACHINE

The elliptical machine is not exactly running, but it's as close as you can get in a knee-saving, nonimpact exercise. It is also an excellent recovery exercise that has the additional advantage of allowing you to use it in an arm-centric, leg-centric, or equally mixed manner. Studies have found the elliptical to have similar VO_2 max development and maintenance to running and stairstepping, but its effect on running performance has not yet been tested.

CROSS-COUNTRY SKIING

This all-body, nonimpact exercise is often said to be the world's single best aerobic exercise; studies have shown that VO_2 max development with cross-country skiing is almost identical to that of running. Other studies have shown that elite skiers have the highest values of VO_2 max of all athletes. Because both arms and legs are used simultaneously, cross-country skiing can stress the heart like no other activity,

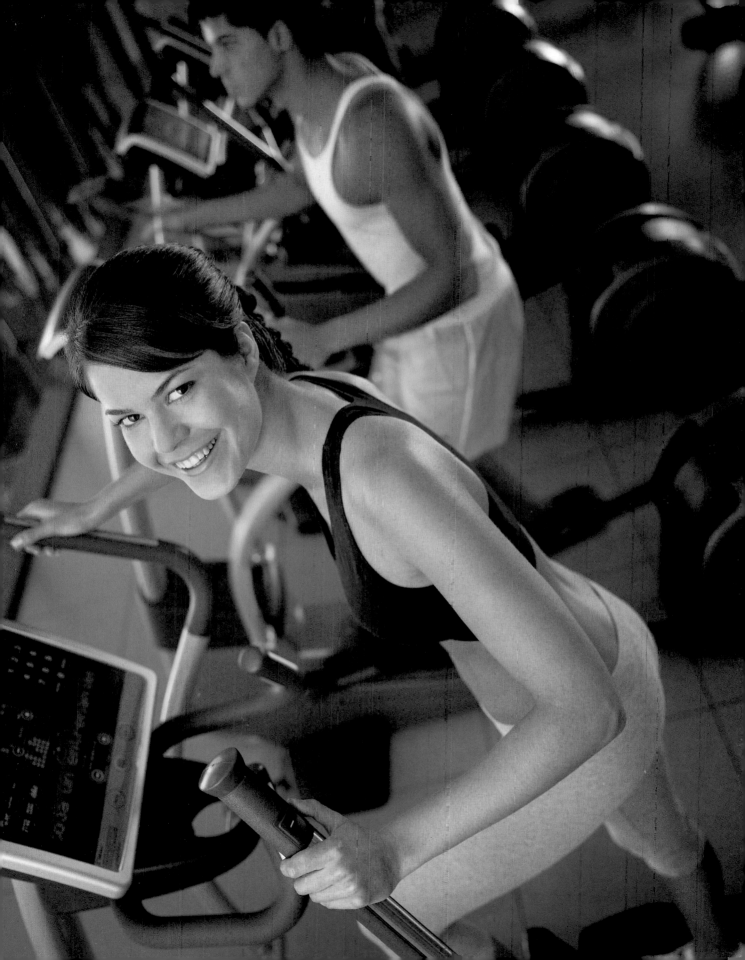

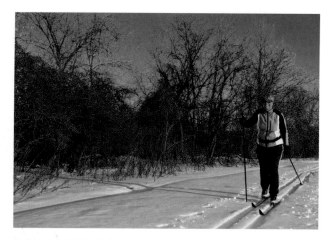

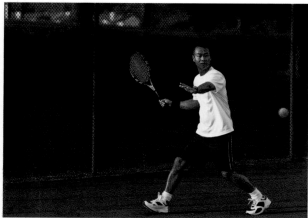

including running. Like the elliptical, however, its specific effect on running performance is not known. A super glute strengthener, cross-country skiing is a great way to get out and train in the winter; the trouble is convenience, as relatively few people have access to cross-country skiing areas. My advice is to take it easy the first time, as you will stress muscles that are underutilized in running, such as your hip flexors.

TENNIS

Surprised? You won't be after you do it, and you sweat like a marathoner in Manila. Although racquet sports are not aerobic per se, the quick-reaction time, fast-rotational forces required, the lateral coordination, and mano a mano skill set that these sports require is, in a way, everything that running isn't. And it gives you a chance to take on a real opponent, not just yourself.

ROWING

Using an ergometer (rowing machine) provides great all-body, calorie-burning cross-training for runners because it's the only no-impact cardio exercise besides swimming that works all four limbs and all the major muscle groups (back, torso, arms, and legs) at once. Done right, rowing blasts your heart and lungs in a safe way, which is easier said than done. Be aware that a proper rowing technique can be hard to master, and an improper technique can hurt your back. Many people are surprised to find that about 70 percent of the rowing motion comes from the legs, with the arm pull taking over only after the legs are nearly fully extended. Here are the steps in a proper rowing technique, as shown opposite:

1. Lean back from your hips while pushing backward with your legs and torso.
2. Keep your arms straight ahead and relaxed until your legs are almost straight, and then flow into an arm pull to finish the motion, pushing your shoulder blades together as you move all the way backward.
3. Try to keep your back straight and don't let it roll forward as you pull. The motion is complete when your elbows pass just behind your chest and the handle is roughly 1 inch (2.5 cm) away from your belly button.
4. Then you will return to the starting position in a mirror image motion and do it all over again.

STRENGTH TRAINING BOOSTS STRENGTH AND BUILDS VO$_2$ MAX

Runners underutilize weight lifting, and some even scorn this form of exercise. "My legs get plenty of work already," some say. "Too much muscle will slow me down," others say. These people are missing the point.

In terms of health, strong muscles are more functional and safer than smaller, weaker ones. They help aerobic performance by increasing your oxygen-processing capacity and providing the strength to push through headwinds and hills. On top of that, big muscles keep you young, helping ward off an aging-related muscle shrinkage that strikes

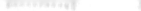

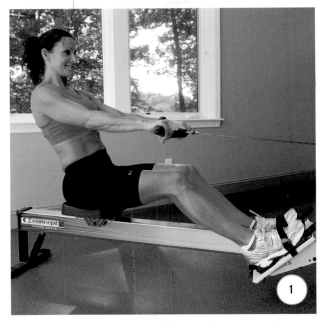

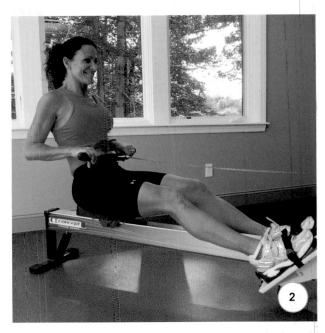

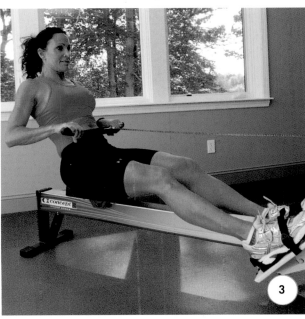

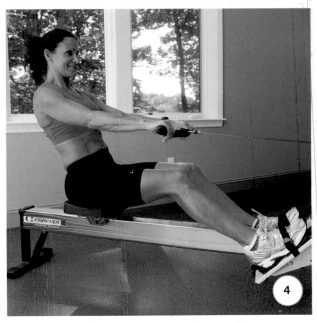

everyone past the age of thirty-five—muscle mass disappears at an average rate of 1 percent per year beginning in your thirties. The steady-state running that most of us do does nothing to stem that decline, even in your legs (unless you do high-intensity intervals and hill work; see Chapter 6 for more details).

The one reliable method for stemming the 1 percent annual decline in muscle mass is weight training. But that doesn't mean merely grabbing a 5 lb. (2.3 kg) dumbbell and doing ten easy biceps curls. Muscle size and strength improve more with more stress. It's officially known as the Stress Adaptation Principle: The harder and faster you push, the stronger you get.

Lifting weights is good for everyone of every age. But for maximum benefit, you must go into the gym the same way you do when you train for a race: with a plan.

STRENGTH-TRAINING RULE 1: DO TWO OR THREE SETS OF HEAVY WEIGHT TO FAILURE

Why lift weights at all if you don't do it hard enough to get stronger? The next time you go to the gym, observe how many people are actually pushing hard. The rule of muscle building is "No strain, no gain." You must work hard enough to set off alarm bells that will alert your brain to send in reinforcements that will strengthen you for the next time, and you do this by going to "failure"—the point at which you can push no more without breaking your form.

Therefore, whether you use dumbbells, barbells, or weight machines, your tenth rep should be a struggle. If you can do an eleventh rep, add more weight. Note: If you use bodyweight exercises such as push-ups, add a weighted belt or increase maximum quantity. To warm up properly and safely, do your first set at lesser weights and more reps, and then go heavier and to failure for the next set or two.

STRENGTH-TRAINING RULE 2: HIT THE WHOLE BODY

Every muscle of the body deteriorates when ignored. A strong upper body contributes to leg speed. A strong back helps you maintain upright form and a good arm swing. Pulling exercises, such as pull-ups and rows, are often ignored but are key to a strong back and help balance out a frequent overemphasis on front-side muscles developed by pushing exercises such as bench presses, chest presses, and push-ups. As in all sports, runners need a strong core, developed not only by a variety of ab exercises, but also by their back-side counterpart, the back extension. Dips are great for working the triceps, balancing the biceps worked by pull-ups and curls. Remember: Steady-state running alone does not stop age-related muscle-mass shrinkage.

STRENGTH-TRAINING RULE 3: MOVE THE WEIGHTS FAST

You don't move slowly in real life, so why move weights in the gym slowly? To build speed, size, and power in every muscle do what pro and college trainers tell their athletes: Go Fast. A caveat: Do it under control with good form so that you don't injure yourself. Explosive movements, although good for you because they rebuild the fast-twitch muscle fibers that we often ignore, can injure you if they take your body by surprise.

Why worry about fast-twitch muscle fibers? First, they keep us safe; giving us the quick reactions we need to dodge rocks on the trail or not trip over errant vacuum-cleaner cords. Next, they deteriorate at a faster rate than slow-twitch muscle fibers, mainly because we use them less often. During running, we mainly use fast-twitch muscles when sprinting, and how often do nontrack runners do that? The bottom line is that well-maintained fast-twitch fibers will make you faster at all running distances and make you safer and healthier in all aspects of life.

If you think you're too old to hit the gym, be aware that pushing heavy weights fast works for all athletes of all ages.

STRENGTH-TRAINING RULE 4: DON'T FORGET THE CALVES, BUTT, HAMSTRINGS, AND HIP FLEXORS

Runners should pay particular attention to a few overlooked muscles. Since calves are so important to running (for shock absorption and push-off), strength-train them with rapid body-weight toe raises on the edge of steps and curbs and heavy weight on calf machines.

Also, don't overly focus on the quadriceps and forget the glutes, hamstrings, and hip flexors. Glutes, the largest muscles in the body, add power and help maintain your posture and running form. Strong quadriceps need to be opposed by strong hamstrings for balance, while strong hip flexors give you range of motion.

Don't have access to a gym? The single best exercise that stimulates all of the aforementioned muscles is the lunge.

STRENGTH-TRAINING RULE 5: DON'T WASTE TIME BETWEEN EXERCISES; PAIR NONCONFLICTING EXERCISES OR USE A CIRCUIT

Here's one surefire way for runners to minimize their time in the gym: Cut out the down time between exercises.

Instead of standing around for sixty seconds in between sets of leg extensions to catch your breath, use that minute to do a nonconflicting exercise, such as a chest press. Do pairs or triplets of nonoverlapping exercises. Follow a bench press, a pushing exercise which works the chest, with a seated row, a pulling exercise which works the back. In this way, one rests as the other is worked, eliminating downtime. This is the idea behind circuit training, which lets you string a dozen nonconflicting exercises together in one circuit, such as dips, calf raises, pull-ups/lat pulls, squats, chest presses, leg extensions, rows, hamstring curls, bicycle sit-ups, biceps curls, overhead presses/handstand push-ups, and back extensions. By the time you finish the loop, you're ready for the second and third circuits.

Proximity is key. If you'll end up wasting time switching from one exercise to another, break the big circuit into smaller mini-circuits that are in the same neighborhood.

STRENGTH-TRAINING RULE 6: EASE INTO IT AND ALLOW FORTY-EIGHT HOURS OF RECOVERY TIME BETWEEN WORKOUTS

Although you need intensity to get results, you should start slow to be safe. Do fewer, lighter-weight reps on your first set (to warm up), take more recovery time (rest and sleep) between workouts, and gradually build up over a good month, after which you can start doing real resistance training without losing time to massive muscle soreness from doing too much, too soon. Since muscle fibers need at least forty-eight hours to recover from a hard workout, don't lift two days in a row. In fact, for best recovery, alternate heavy and light workouts.

Muscles learn. If you do the same exercises all the time, the exercises get easier. A movement that initially took ten muscle fibers to move soon takes nine fibers, and then eight. To keep firing all the fibers, you need to add more weight and/or change the exercises you do every couple of months. Mix it up. At a macro level, lift heavier weights for fewer reps (eight or seven to failure) for a month, and then switch to more, lighter-weight reps (twelve to fifteen to failure). At a micro level, change your technique. Do biceps curls, but change your grip from underhand to overhand, machines to dumbbells.

STRENGTH-TRAINING RULE 7: COOL DOWN WITH A RECOVERY SPIN AND STRETCHING

After you lift weights, your capillaries are dilated, so jump on an easy cardio machine to cool down, and then stretch (see Chapter 5). The bike or elliptical machine allows you to slowly bring your heart rate down. As a runner, you may have a tendency to want to hop on a treadmill, but fight this. You've already blasted your legs with the machines; they don't need any more micro-tears at this point. For the same reason, a hard run the next day is not a good idea; if you must run, consider an easy recovery run on a softer surface, such as a trail, or water running.

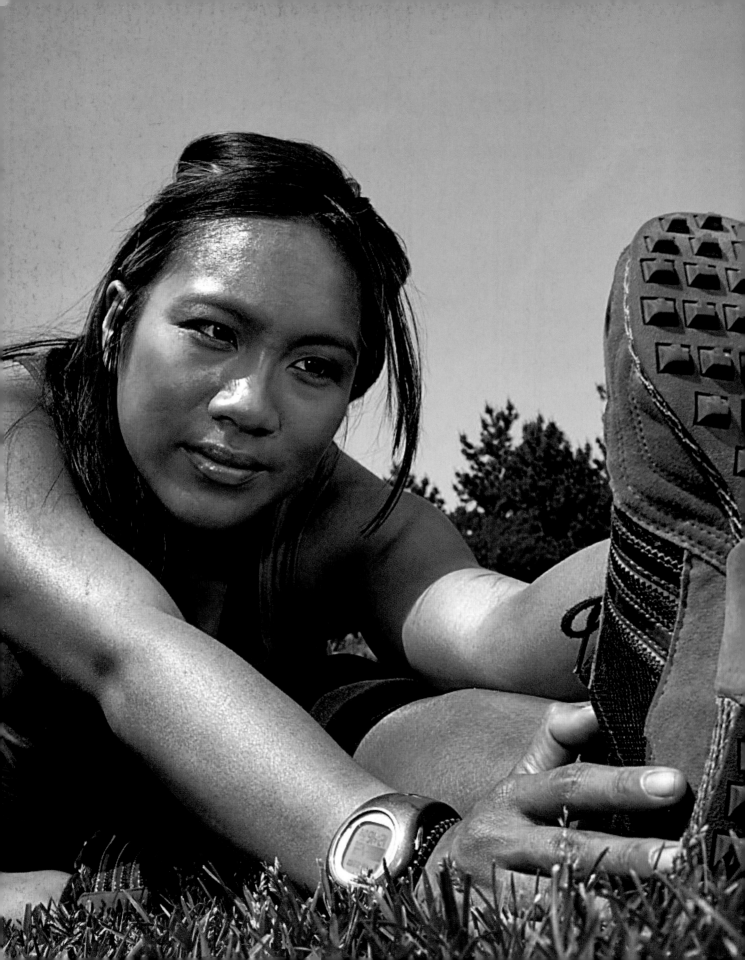

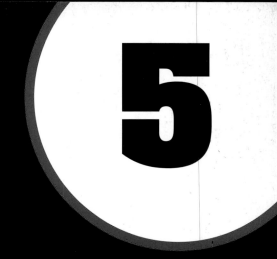

5

>>> # STRENGTH TRAINING, CROSS-TRAINING, AND FLEXIBILITY

LET ME SAY TWO WORDS ABOUT STRETCHING: Do it. In fact, do it a lot. Runners are notoriously tight. According to Bob Anderson, the author of *Stretching*, the flexibility bible that has sold 3.5 million copies and has been translated into twenty-eight languages since it was written in 1975, this tightness is the rare malady that any runner can completely reverse. He says the immediate benefits of stretching are too good to pass up:

- Faster speed, due to more efficient biomechanics
- More force, due to the increased leverage of lengthened muscles
- Faster post-run recovery

THE TWELVE RULES OF STRETCHING

All runners know they should stretch, but hardly anyone really knows how to do it right. Here's how to get the most out of stretching.

WARM UP FIRST

Before any stretching, do a few minutes of easy running to make sure your muscles are appropriately warmed up. Stretching cold, tight muscles is probably worse than not stretching at all.

RELAX

If possible, stretch passively, meaning stretch while lying down on the floor, not standing. Relax the muscle by taking it out of a weight-bearing and/or body stabilization position prior to the stretch. Generally, it's harder to relax a muscle while it is under tension.

TOSS THE TOE-TOUCH

Never reach over to touch your toes from a standing position. The lower back is concave; this move makes it convex. "Your back ligaments are already stretched out by cycling, and they don't need to be stretched more," says Carl Foster "A guy with a discectomy isn't finding enlightenment."

TAKE IT SLOW

Use the subsiding tension principle. Move slowly into the stretch and allow for tension to register before adjusting your intensity. Rapid stretching can stimulate the muscle to tighten up rather than lengthen. Hold stretches for fifteen to thirty seconds.

BREATHE EASY

Be in a position in which you can breathe slowly and rhythmically while holding your stretches. Exhale slowly as you extend to the endpoint of the stretch. As you exhale, your diaphragm and thoracic-cavity muscles should be relaxing, thus promoting a more effective relaxation of the target muscles.

FEEL NO PAIN

Stretch to the limit of movement, not the point of pain. This is referred to as the endpoint of the stretch. If the stretch yields pain, back off the movement and make sure the stretching technique is correct. It may be necessary to try another position or a different stretching exercise (or method).

FOCUS ON ONE MUSCLE AT A TIME

Focus only on the muscle or muscles involved in the stretch, minimizing the movement of other body parts. Systematically stretch each major muscle and muscle group. Don't try to rush by attempting to stretch several muscles at once. You'll get a substandard stretch and you'll risk injury.

ALTER THE ANGLE

Stretch the muscles in various positions, as this may improve the overall range of movement at the joint. For example, to stretch your hamstrings from different angles, switch hands; first, grab your right toe with your right hand, and then switch and grab your right toe with your left hand. This will give you more of a cross-body movement that will stretch the hamstring more on its lateral side, along with the IT band.

HIT 'EM ALL

Stretch all of your major muscle groups as well as the opposing muscle groups. For example, after your biceps, hit your triceps; do the same with your abdominals and lower back, and quads and hamstrings.

DON'T BLOW IT OFF

Stretch after each vigorous workout.

DO IT ANYTIME

You can stretch before you work out, after you work out—indeed, any time of the day or night.

- **Before:** Stretch right after you warm up, and within forty-five minutes of a workout or race.

- **After:** Try to stretch within forty-five minutes after a workout, while you're warm, to aid circulation and recovery, and correct gross imbalances. The simple rule is to keep the total stretching to fifteen minutes, and probably no more than sixty seconds for any one stretch.
- **Anytime:** Bob Anderson (see below) likes to stretch before he goes to bed, which promotes a functional remodeling of connective tissue to create a stronger infrastructure. But make sure to be warm and supple before you stretch.

THE TOP TEN STRETCHES FOR RUNNERS

Bob Anderson recommends that you find four or five stretches that really help you and do them several times per day, including at bedtime. He recommends that you choose from the following menu of ten basic stretches to maintain range of motion from toe to head.

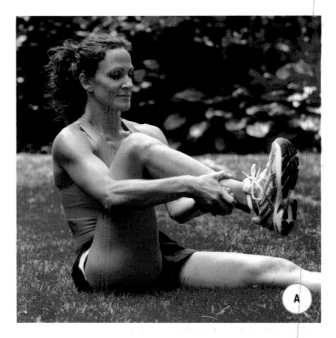

ANKLE ROTATION A

The ankle is important for overall flexibility. To keep it loose, sit on the floor with your legs spread apart, and then grab one ankle with both hands and rotate it clockwise and counterclockwise through a complete range of motion with slight resistance provided. This rotary motion of the ankle helps to gently stretch tight ligaments and improve circulation. Repeat ten to twenty times in each direction. Do both ankles.

SITTING CALF AND HAMSTRING STRETCH B

This movement stretches the lower leg's rear muscles and the area behind the knee. Sit upright with one leg straight ahead and the other leg bent at the knee, with the bottom of the foot on your bent leg resting flat against the inner thigh of your outstretched leg. If you are not very flexible, point your toes toward your body, and lean at your waist toward the extended foot until you feel a stretch in the back of your

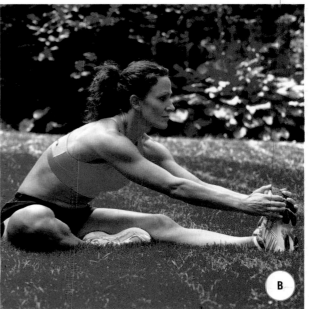

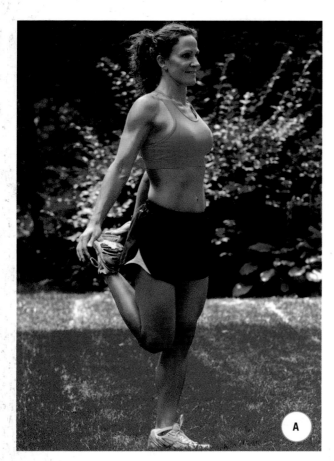

A

knee. Hold this position for ten to fifteen seconds.

If you are flexible, assume the same position, but reach out with the same-side hand, grab the back of your toes, and pull them toward you. Keep your head up and your back as straight as possible.

OPPOSITE HAND/OPPOSITE FOOT QUAD STRETCH Ⓐ

Lying on your side or standing, hold the top of your right foot with your left hand and gently pull your heel toward your buttocks. The knee bends at a natural angle when you hold your foot with the opposite hand. This is good to use in knee rehabilitation and by those with problem knees. Hold each leg in this position for thirty seconds.

SPINAL TWIST: LOWER BACK AND HAMSTRINGS Ⓑ

Although Anderson warns that this stretch is difficult for the average person to do, it is highly beneficial for the back. Sit on the floor with your right leg straight ahead. Bend your left leg, cross your left foot over to the outside of your upper-right thigh, just above your knee. During the stretch, use your elbow to keep your left leg stationary with controlled pressure to the inside. With your left hand resting behind you, slowly turn your head to look over your left shoulder and at the same time rotate your upper body toward your left hand and arm. This should stretch your lower back and side of hip. Hold for fifteen seconds. Do both sides.

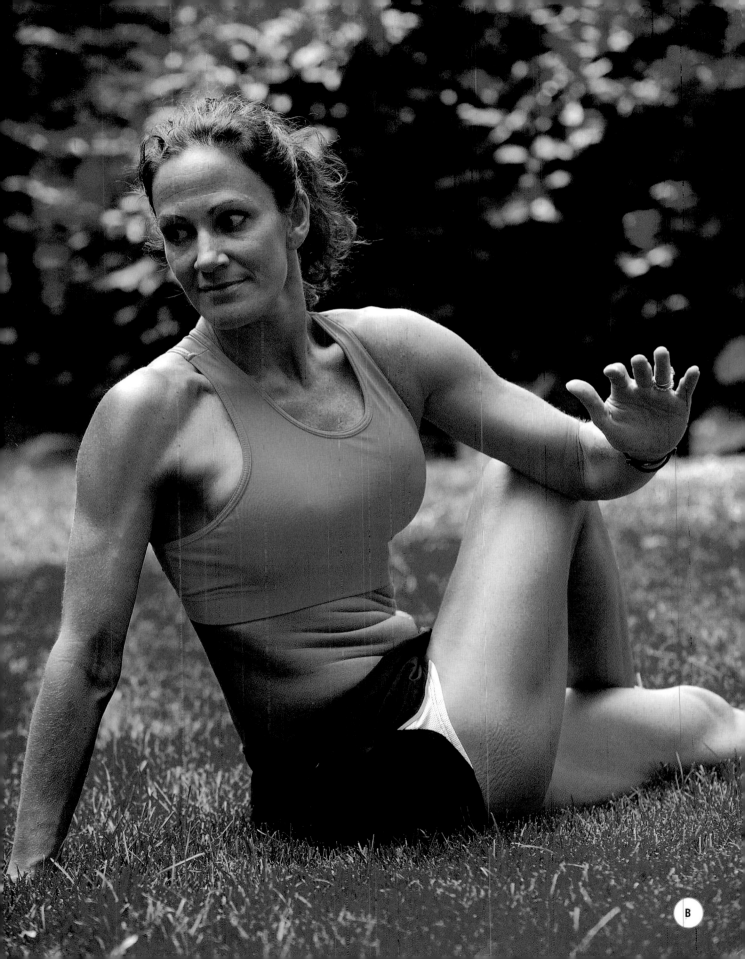

B

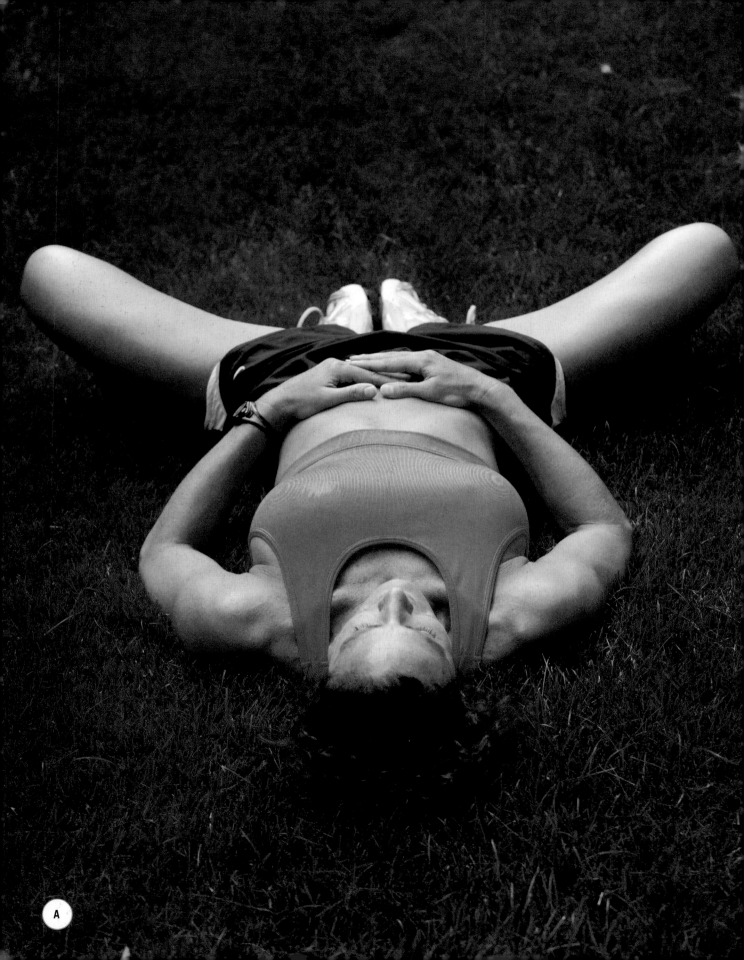

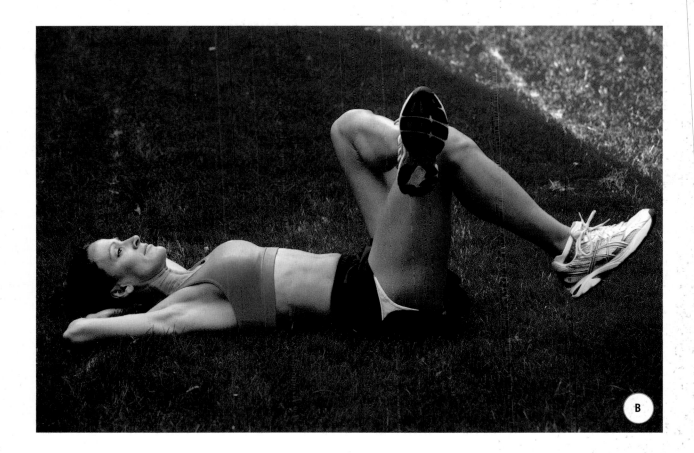

GROIN AND BACK STRETCH Ⓐ

This comfortable stretch is an easy, safe way to stretch an area that is often tight and hard to relax: the groin. It also flattens your lower back, helping counteract a hump. Lie on your back with your knees bent, the soles of your feet together, and your hands resting on your stomach. Let your knees hang down toward the floor, allowing gravity to stretch your groin. By contrast, people often sit up and perform a groin stretch by leaning forward with a rounded-back torso that is hard on the back ligaments.

SECRETARY STRETCH FOR LOWER BACK AND HIPS Ⓑ

Here's another stretch for the back, which also happened to be great for people with sciatic pain. Lying on your back with your knees up in a sit-up position, interlace your fingers behind your head and lift your left leg over your right leg. From here, pivot your left leg to the right, pulling your right leg toward the floor until you feel a good stretch along the side of your hip and lower back. Stretch and relax. Keep your upper back, shoulders, and elbows flat on the floor. Hold for twenty to thirty seconds. Repeat the stretch for the other side.

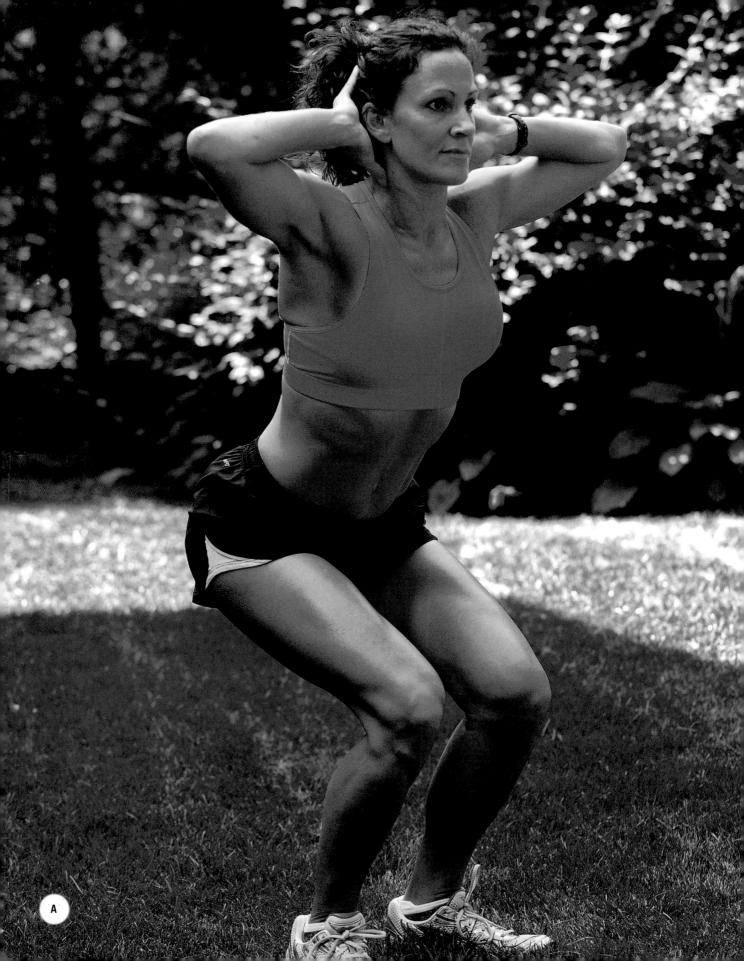

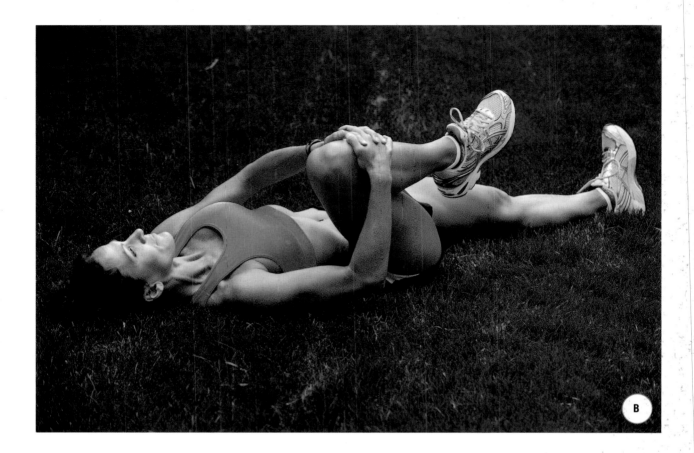

B

THE SAIGON SQUAT

"If I had one stretch to do, this would be it for keeping overall muscle and joint flexibility," says Anderson. "It's the most natural position in human history—squatting to relieve yourself in a floor-pit toilet." The squat stretches everything from the mid-section down, including the ankles, Achilles tendons, groin, lower back, and hips. Anderson is fond of pointing out that the squat taxes humans much more than the seated-position Western toilet, which is why rural Asians usually have better postures and livelier steps than their occidental counterparts.

The squat is simple to perform: With your feet shoulder-width apart and pointed out to about a fifteen-degree angle, and with your heels on the ground, bend your knees and squat down. Hold for thirty seconds. If you have ultra-tight Achilles tendons, you can't balance with flat feet, and you generally have trouble staying in this position, hold on to something for support. If you have knee problems, discontinue this stretch at the first sign of pain.

WILLIAMS' FLEXION HAMSTRING STRETCH B

Considered very relaxing and safe after a run, this easy stretch is great for pelvis flexibility, hip flexors, back, and circulation (because it gets the foot above the heart). To do it, lie on your back, keeping your back flat, and draw one knee into your chest by pulling it in from the back of the knee; repeat with the other leg. For variation, pull your knee toward your opposite shoulder.

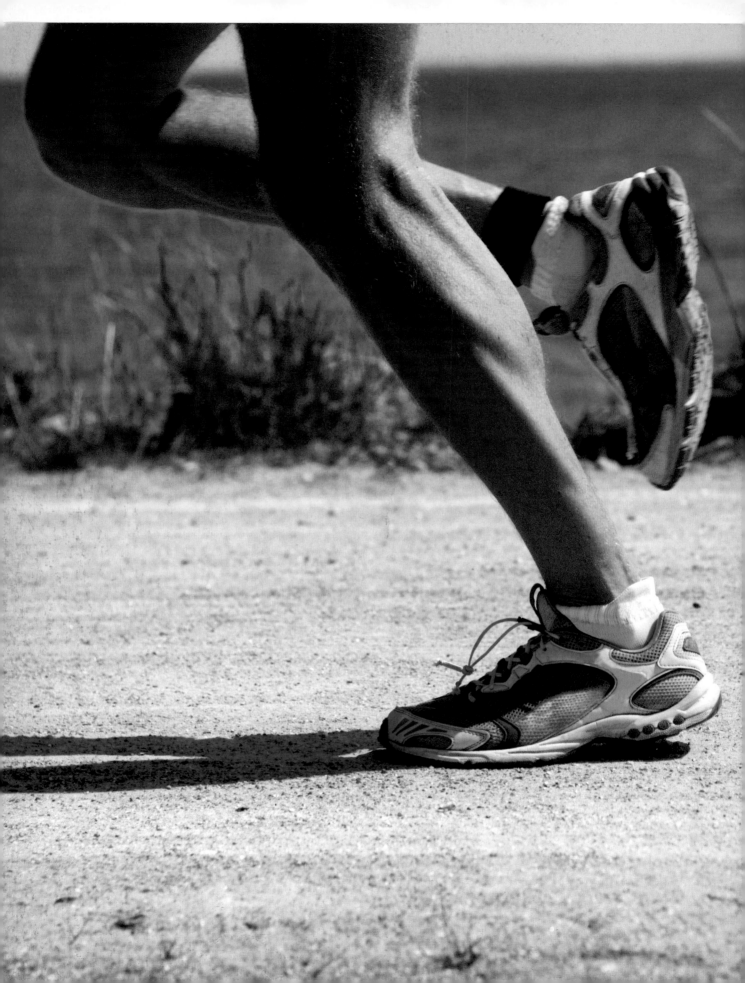

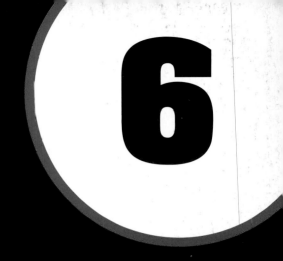

CHOOSING A VARIETY OF SURFACES AND LOCATIONS: STRONGER, FASTER RUNNING BY TRAINING ON DIFFERENT SURFACES

FOR MOTIVATION AND INJURY REDUCTION, the best place to run is the path less traveled. Out of habit, most people run the same route over and over, year after year, but that's not such a good idea. This chapter will explain why it's far better to run on a variety of different surfaces—roads, hills, treadmills, tracks, and dirt trails—that together will serve to stimulate your mind and body and make your running more fun, safer, and more effective.

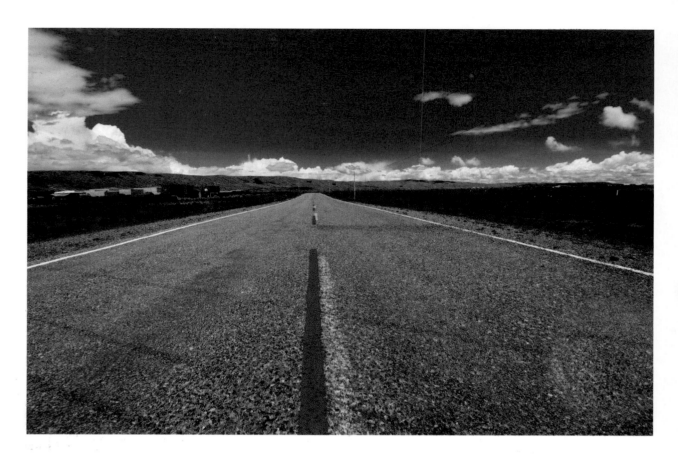

THE ROADS: STREET-SMART SAFETY RULES

Bursting out your front door and running on the local roads surrounding your home—what most of us do most of the time—is hard to beat for convenience and efficiency, but that doesn't mean you can't do it better. Not all roads are created equal; some are better for running, some worse. In general, stay away from concrete, aim for straight, well-lit, traffic-free byways, and keep yourself highly visible and aware of the sights and sounds of your environment. Here's more detail:

- **Avoid the sidewalk.** Getting off the street to avoid auto traffic seems like a good idea at first—until you realize that the concrete on sidewalks is harder and less maintained than the asphalt on roads. The hardness subjects your legs to an increased pounding that can make you susceptible to injury; in general, go for the softer surface. The typically poorer maintenance of sidewalks—often cracked and unleveled by tree roots, plus littered with parked and backing-out cars, children's toys, and pedestrians—can made the sidewalk a dangerous obstacle course that has you swerving out of the way and jumping on and off curbs. Run in the streets.

- **Beware the camber.** Roads that are highly cambered (arched) from center to side, which aids drainage, can throw off your form by putting your legs at different levels and unbalancing your body for long periods of time. The only level spot is the dead center of the road, which isn't a safe place. Run on flatter roads, bike paths, and parks. Although the grass of a park or the periphery of a playing field may have uneven spots, it usually won't have camber issues.

- **Make yourself visible.** You can reduce the risk of getting hit by a car by running against traffic, wearing reflective gear, avoiding winding roads, and not crossing intersections.

- **Go against traffic.** Drivers are distracted, are rushed, and don't expect slow vehicles or people to be sharing the road, so try to get their attention by going against the flow. Running against traffic may make it easier for you to make eye contact and for drivers to move over.

- **Beware of winding ways.** Curves are a real danger, as they prevent drivers from seeing you until the last minute. So are intersections, which expose you to unaware cross-traffic. So, make eye contact when you cross. Take it easy on yourself by choosing a route that limits road crossings, making as many left turns as possible.

- **Be safe at sundown.** Limit running at dusk, when the light is low but many drivers don't have their headlights on and often are driving tired. If you like to run at night (which we don't recommend), wear gear with reflective patches and carry ID in case of an accident.

- **Look for minimal traffic, wide shoulders, and low speeds.** Avoid busy roads with no shoulders or room to escape oncoming traffic. Have an escape route: a sidewalk or ditch that you can use to avoid being hit.

- **Hike the headphones.** People swear by their iPods, but music players can be hazardous to your health. If they stop you from hearing cars, you'll respond to danger more slowly. If music is a must, turn the volume down as low as possible to stay aware of your surroundings.

- **Don't space out.** Look where you're going—not down, but forward. This will ensure that you see any danger coming your way.

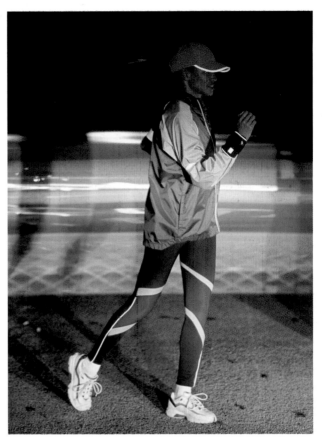

Wear light-colored reflective clothing when running at night.

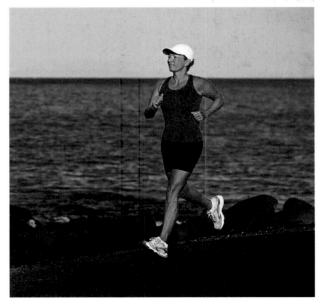

Run against traffic and on quiet roads. Look straight ahead and stay alert.

CHOOSE GOOD RUNNING ROUTES

Once you've chosen an area that has a good surface, favorable terrain, and minimal traffic, now what? Some people like to explore as they run, checking out different neighborhoods and deliberately getting lost, while others feel more comfortable with a well-laid-out plan.

There are a variety of options for the latter, starting with Map My Run, an Internet route-mapping website filled with routes input by real runners (see www.mapmyrun.com). You can find out exactly how long a run near your home is and what the terrain will be like.

GPS leader Garmin is behind Garmin Connect (http://connect.garmin.com/), a free service that connects you with routes. Getting excellent reviews is MotionBased.com (http://motionbased.com/), which covers cities all over the United States. Just type in your ZIP Code and it whisks you to a community forum of local members who discuss their favorite routes.

USE GPS TO MAP YOUR ROUTE

With the proliferation of GPS-enabled devices and mapping services, it's easy to plan a route to take, or find out where, how fast, and how far you went. Check Chapter 11 for details on the Apple iPhone upbeat workouts, iPod, Body Bugg, accelerometers, SmartFabrics and other technologies that can provide lots of route data and feedback. On the horizon is a wave of new innovations, one of which is A Network Tiny (ANT), a new wireless sensor network chip technology housed in cell phones, watches, and other devices that allows them all to communicate with one another.

HILLS: TAKING YOUR RUNNING TO NEW HEIGHTS

Some runners hate the hills, but the benefits of running them are so great that you should learn to love them. Hills are among the best training tools for improving your stamina/endurance, speed, and muscular power. They'll make you a better, fitter, mentally tougher runner who finishes higher in your age group at races, and can add a level of fun that is just not possible on the flats. And they do it without all the steady-state pounding of flat-land running, so they are safer for your joints and connective tissue.

Hill running is so good because it is more than aerobics; it's also strength training—you're working against the forces of gravity. In fact, some coaches favor hill running over other forms of weight-bearing exercise for runners because it builds muscular power while targeting the muscles you actually use in running. Going against gravity makes the buttocks, hamstrings, quads, and calves work even harder, much like speedwork, which it enhances. And with the reduced pounding—confirmed in a Nike study which found that hill running subjects the body to just 85 percent of the shock of running the flats—you can do hill training more regularly than conventional speedwork without getting as beat up.

The increased power derived from hill training will also translate to increased stamina. If you follow our hill-running method, which aims for the same natural rhythm that you use in the flats, you'll keep the pace through the ups and downs of a race or a training run. You'll run through your periods of exhaustion, aware of it but not focusing on it, due to the mental and physical toughness developed on the climbs.

HILL TRAINING METHOD: BUILD UP GRADUALLY

We recommend that you incorporate hill training into your training as soon as you get into a comfortable running routine on the flats. But ease into it; don't try to do too many hills at once, which may leave you burned out, intimidated, and injured. Initially, add some rolling hills and see how your body responds. Like all the advice we give in this book, keep it in moderation.

After you climb some hills, carefully follow up and evaluate how you feel. Reflect on your body's performance by monitoring your heart rate, or Rating of Perceived Exertion (RPE), or the talk test, all mentioned earlier and discussed in more detail in Chapter 7. If you are finding that you are out of breath or have overexerted yourself, keep your larger goals in mind and don't overexert yourself just for one little hill. Build up gradually until the hills are part of your routine, or run on the flats and walk up the hills to get your muscle fibers used to this kind of work.

Once you are comfortable on the hills, there are all sorts of interesting ways to incorporate them into your training. One favorite is to drive to a hill and run it over and over. This is an efficient workout that, when you become too exerted, allows you to get into your car and drive home after a time-efficient strength and cardiovascular workout.

Six Ways to Downshift Your Way Up a Hill

There are many ways to climb a hill, but only one best method, according to our research. Cyclists know that the first thing to do to prepare for an ascent is to downshift their gears. Well, runners should do the same thing: downshift mentally and physically. Here's what that means:

- **Release all tension.** When you're running toward a hill, don't tense up or resist it. Save your resistance for gravity—that's where you're going to need it. Resist the urge to speed up, gaining momentum for your heroic ascent. Do a mental check on your body. Release neck and shoulder tension. Unclench those fists. Save it for the hill.

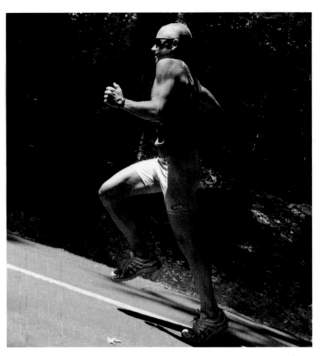

Good running form: When running hills, relax the body and shorten the stride. Engage your arms to increase your speed.

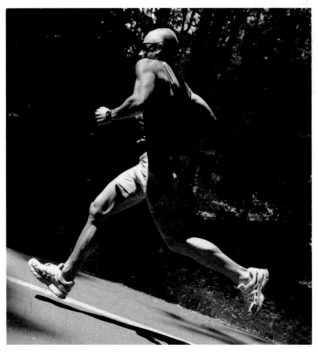

Incorrect hill form: This runner is taking long strides as if to "power" his way up the hill; this will result in exhaustion. Don't let your foot get out in front of your head.

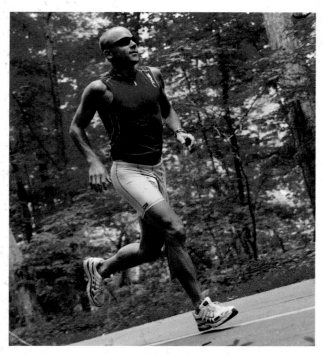

Good form: When running hills, the upper body should be relaxed and slightly forward. Keep the feet under the hips and center of gravity.

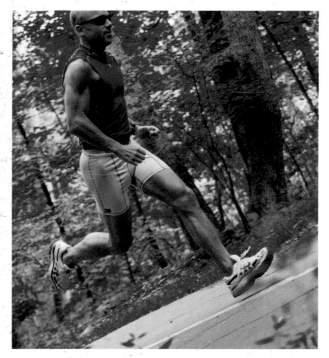

Incorrect form: This runner is striding far in front of his center of gravity and holding his arms tight against his sides.

- **Shorten your stride and slow down.** Once the ascent begins, physically downshift. Gradually shorten your stride, focusing on the power that comes with each lift. Concentrate on maintaining an even effort as you did on the flats. That's going to mean slowing down. Don't bound; bounding up the hill will result in exhaustion and frustration. Take your time.
- **Be a lean machine.** Lean slightly into the hill, but don't exaggerate the lean too much. A shorter stride allows you to put more power into each step. Always keep your foot under your center of mass, not ahead of it. Think about when you're walking up stairs; your foot is never ahead of your head, which is leaned forward. Don't lift your knees high, as that wastes too much energy. Focus on the lift that comes from your toe-off.
- **Use your arms.** A little-known secret to getting up the hills with less effort is to actively engage your arms. They should act as levers that increase your speed. Focus on them. They should be relaxed just as they are on the flats, but with a more forceful backswing. An exaggerated backswing helps provide lift to the knees. I'm not a biomechanist, but I know what works: On the hills, you use your arms to drive your legs. Don't swing so high that you feel out of alignment or the movement feels forced or unnatural.
- **Keep your head up and your body erect.** Keep your posture straight and gaze ahead. Don't focus on the top of the hill, but do look confidently ahead of yourself; don't hunker down into it. Your goal is to keep up your rhythm and to be as comfortable and natural as possible.
- **Speed up near the top.** After enough focus and energy, the end is near. As the top becomes visible and the hill begins to crest, celebrate by picking up your rhythm. Remember, your goal should be to run as evenly as possible, on any kind of terrain. Use that momentum—that drive and focus—to carry you over the other side, where gravity will become your friend.

▶ Efficient hill-running form. Notice the short stride, slightly forward posture, and strong backswing. The head is up, the gaze straight ahead.

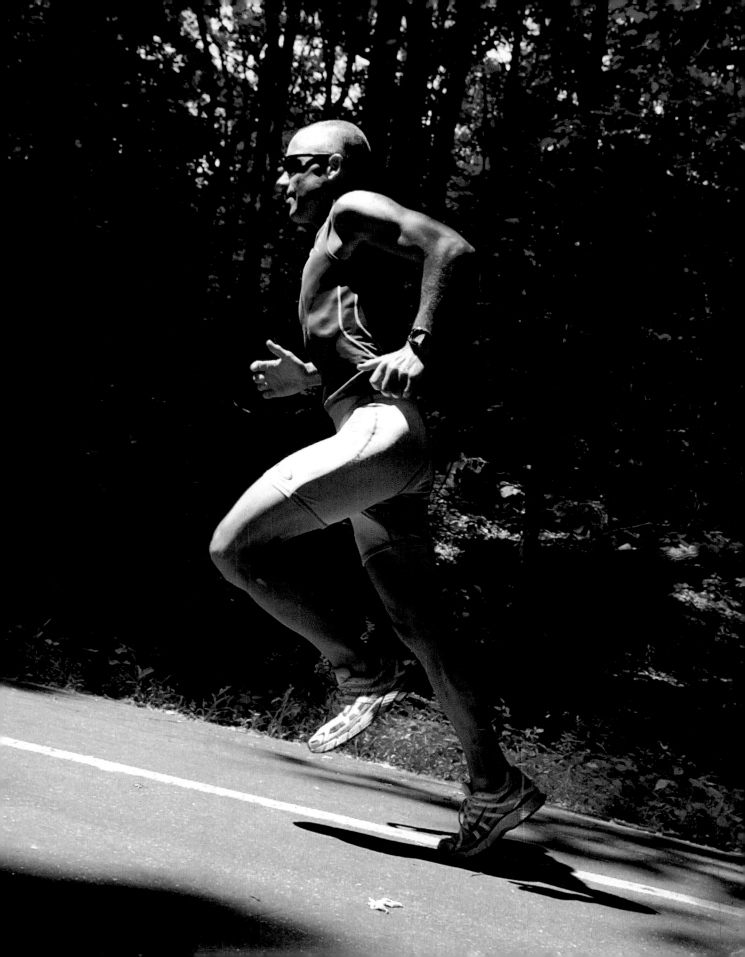

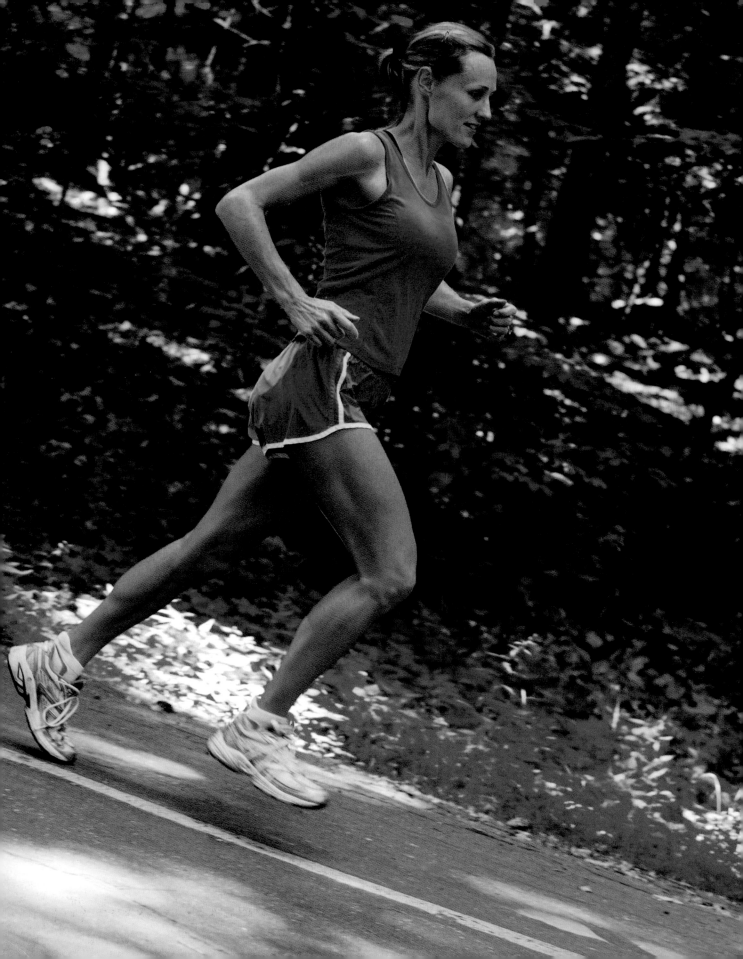

How to "Think" Your Way Up a Hill—No, Really!

The mental side of hill running is a critical part of making it a satisfying experience and doing it well. Proper attitude is key. If you look at a hill as an obstacle, or a foe to be conquered, you may well find the work difficult. John "The Penguin" Bingham writes in his column in *Competitor Magazine*, "Don't fight the hill—be the hill." In other words, you'll be more successful if you think of a hill as an interesting landscape that your body can relax into and be a part of. An effective visualization, according to Bob Glover, esteemed New York Road Runners coach and author, is to imagine yourself ascending effortlessly, as if someone were towing you up the hill.

The bottom line is to not get hung up on how high the hill is or stare at the top and obsess about it. Imagine how great you will feel as you crest it. In fact, if you train on hills, you may look forward to them because you are used to seeing them as challenges and opportunities to succeed. Try to welcome hills, enjoying the sensation of pushing against the forces of gravity.

FIVE WAYS TO MASTER THE DOWNHILL

The downhill is a place to get great gains fast. That's because it's the side that runners spend the least amount of time working on. Get ready to improve quickly.

- **Give in to gravity.** As you approach the crest of the hill at the end of the climb and your pace increases, you'll feel gravity release its hold. Then, as you start your descent, let it work for you, pulling you down the hill. Let gravity do the work and go with it, unless the hill is so steep you feel off-balance.
- **Go low with the flow.** Avoid feeling like you are braking with every step; lean slightly into the hill and enjoy the ride. Keep your feet low to the ground and stay in a controlled flow.

◀ Proper downhill form: The body leans slightly forward and the feet stay close to the ground.

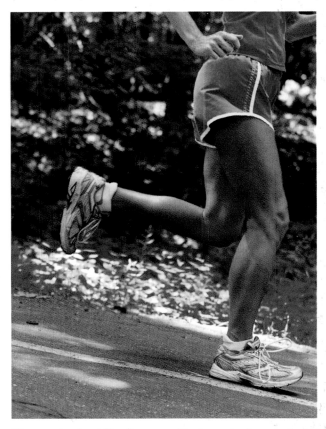

When running downhill, make your stride shorter. Land on your heels, right under your body.

- **Take shorter steps.** Avoid overstriding, which will pound your joints hard with the additional gravity. Land with your heels under you for stability.
- **Do more core work.** Consciously engage your core muscles to make the pounding have less of an impact.
- **Watch out!** Pay attention to obstacles or areas such as gravel where you might slip.
- **Hold your arms out.** Hold your arms slightly out from your body to maintain your balance, as you would while riding a mountain bike downhill.

Downhills can be dangerous and tough on your body; stay light on your feet, feel the flow of the hill, don't overstride, and you will be refreshed and rejuvenated by the time you reach the bottom.

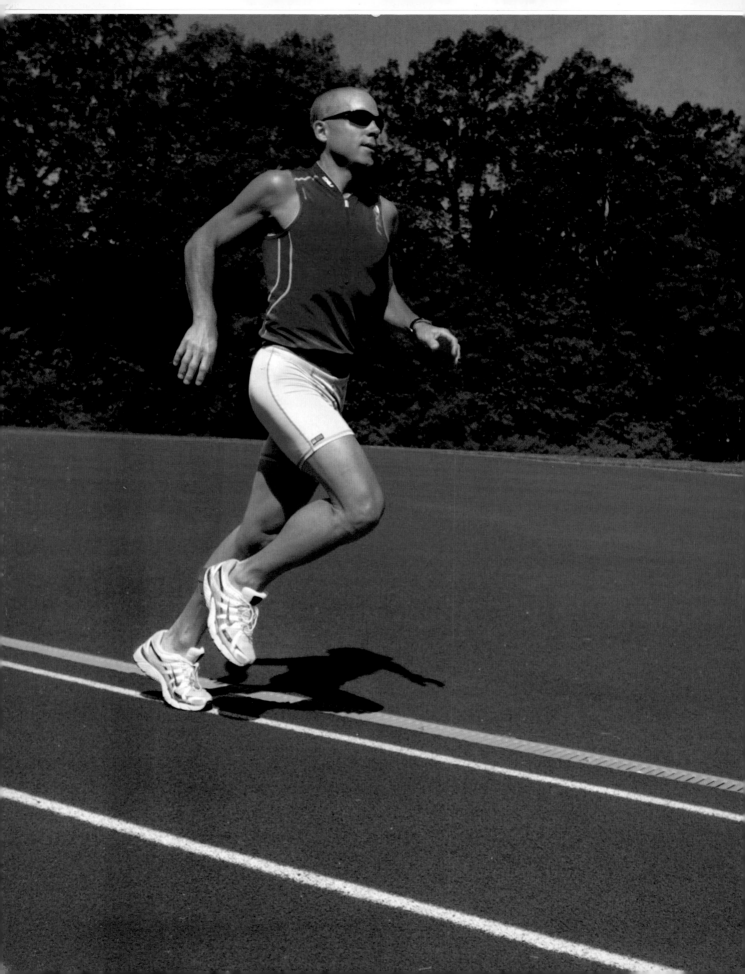

you're not training at the same pace. That convenience extends to running with kids, since you can keep them in sight at all times. You can turn up your headphones to full-blast without a care about personal safety.

Now, the cons:

- **Loop-de-loops can drive you loopy.** Running in circles can be less interesting than running on the roads. Many would find it boring, a drudgery, to do a long-distance run circling a track; it might be advisable to run to the track, looping it for a while, and then run home, before monotony sets in.
- **Locals might see you.** Self-conscious types might prefer not to run in their neighborhood, while others might find it intimidating to run on a track with seasoned runners, even though your pace certainly won't matter to them. After all, they are running for themselves. You are running for you.

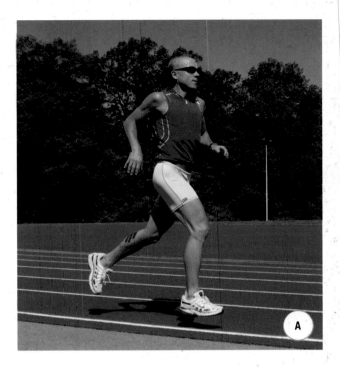

TRACK-RUNNING BASICS

Keep these basics in mind for top-notch track workouts:

- **Go to school.** Finding a track should be easy, as most high schools and colleges, and even some middle schools, have a standard 0.25-mile (400 m) oval.
- **Do the math.** The standard track makes it easy to measure out a mile—four times around the track. Like the treadmill, it will be easy to track improvements in pace because of the similarity of each track run.

- **Change direction or try the outside lane 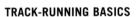.** Although a track has a springier surface than asphalt, the tight turns in a single direction can be hard on your joints. Solution? Change direction whenever the track is empty, or stay in the outside lane to make the turns less sharp and reduce the strain on your body.
- **Avoid the track during a meet.** Know the hours that the track is booked for events. You will not be allowed onto the track while a track meet is in progress.

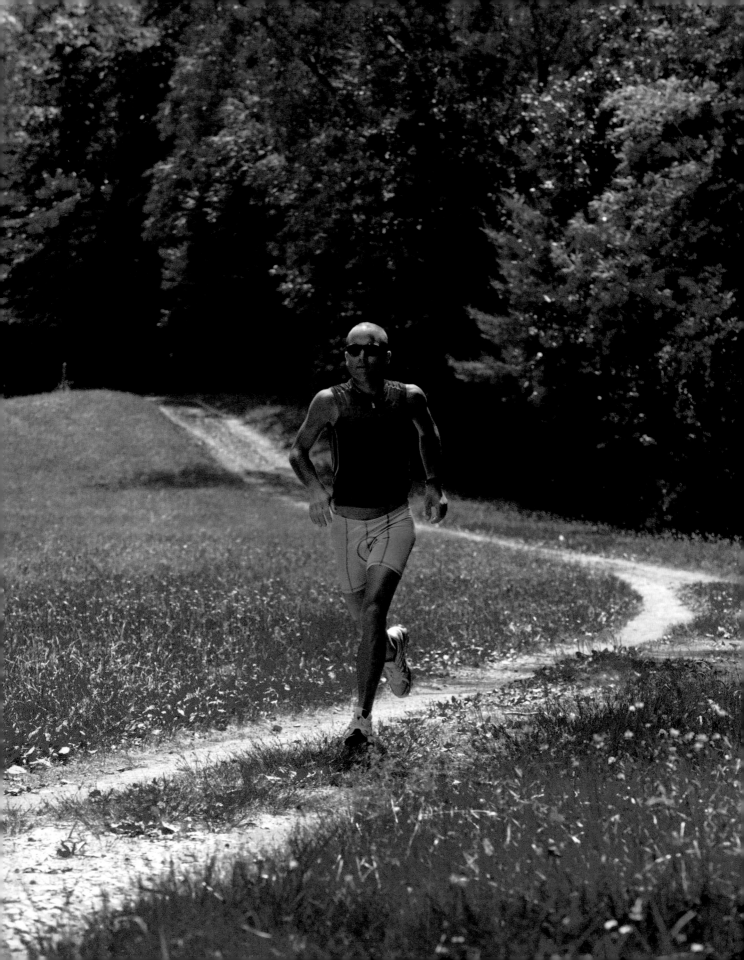

TRAIL RUNNING: WHY YOU NEED TO HIT THE DIRT

Nothing is better for improving foot and leg strength, enhancing overall body stability, and reducing the risk of running injuries than training on trails. Many people who are relatively new to running don't consider running off-road, and that's too bad. Although the unpredictable surface angulation and consistency can seem daunting to someone who has never tried it, those same challenging characteristics have the potential to strengthen your body from the feet up, ramp up your running excitement, and extend your running career.

BENEFITS AND CHALLENGES OF VARIABLE TERRAIN

Running on dirt has some serious benefits:

- **Better workout:** Studies have shown that trail running requires 26 percent more effort than road running because of the constant adjustments and changes in stride that are required. The additional effort you expend means you get more bang for your buck in terms of fitness levels.

- **Improved stability:** These adjustments also mean you will improve stabilization and will become more coordinated.

- **Injury reduction:** Because you need to use your body in a different way, you use different muscles and break the overuse patterns many runners fall into.

But trail running also has some challenges:

- You can't zone out. You must be constantly aware of where your feet are falling—or else you soon may be falling. So, enjoy the scenery, but in small bites. Gaze too long and you may run off a cliff.

- You can't always hammer. The rough terrain may make it difficult to break out into the full speeds that are possible in a road run. You must be constantly mindful of avoiding injury and scanning ahead of you for hazards.

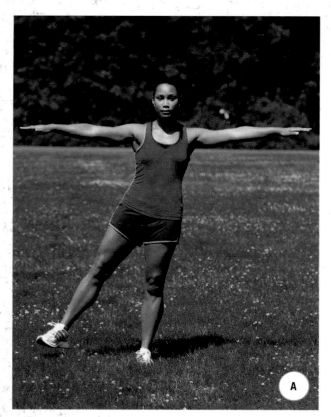

A

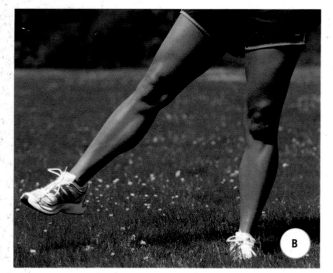

B

BACK-TO-NATURE FORM CHANGES

Although running on natural surfaces such as grass, sand, and trails seems instinctive, all of these can be challenging if you are used to running on the streets. Grass is frequently studded with holes and bumps; the slant of the beach and shifting sands make for an uneven strain on your body; trails almost seem designed to trip you. Here are the form changes you need to make to handle the best that Mother Nature can throw at you:

- Shorten your step length and lift your knees higher to negotiate obstacles in your path.
- Keep your eyes ahead about two steps, looking down for potential hazards.
- Do ankle-strengthening drills **A** **B** **C**. The uneven surfaces on trails inflict more strain and instability on the ankles, which may bother some runners. To get used to this, practice balancing on one leg or on a balance trainer to build up strength in your ankles.

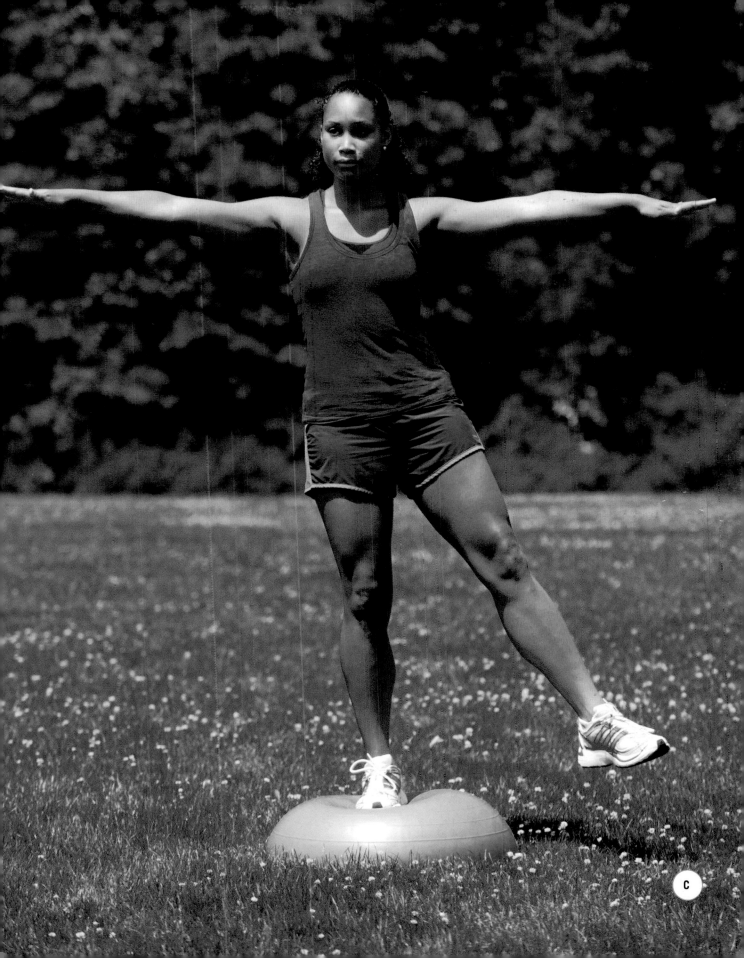

C

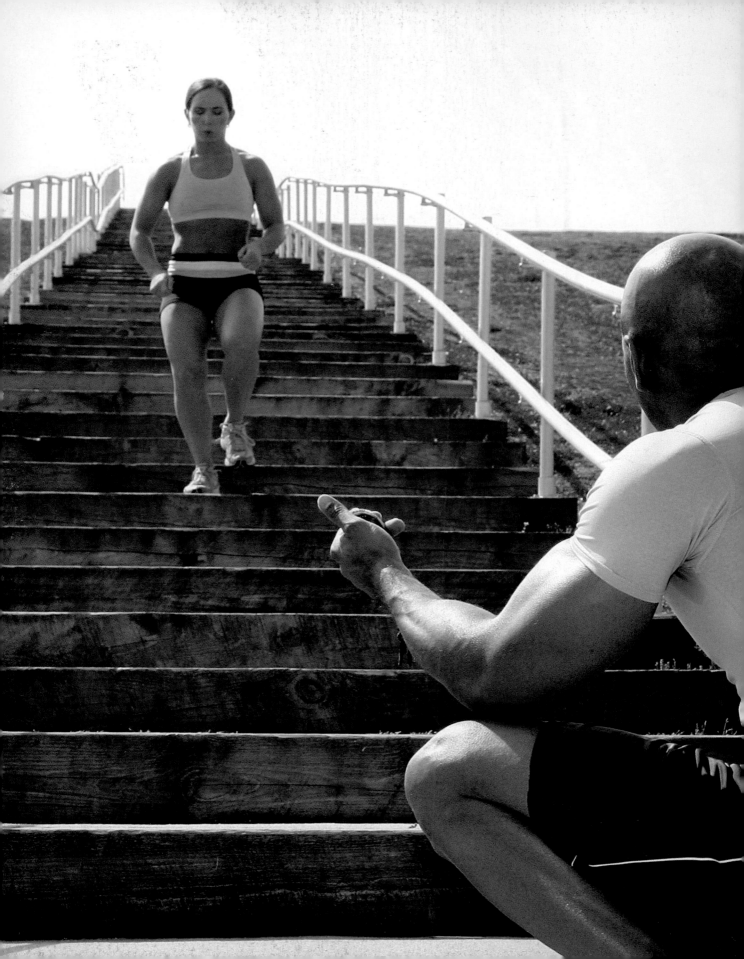

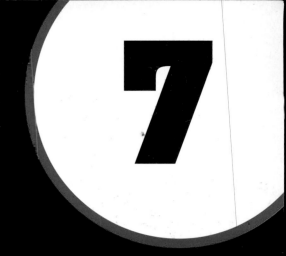

USING SCIENCE FOR BETTER RUNNING: DECADES-LONG RESEARCH FOR OPTIMAL TRAINING

CARL HAS HAD A FRONT-ROW SEAT—sometimes the driver's seat—on the long, scientific road to an optimal universal training methodology. Obsessed with improving his running times as a youth, Carl has spent his professional life working with some the world's best-known running coaches and theorists on a quest for improving athletic performance. Here he connects the dots of running research, looking back at how far we've come in our knowledge of training, and examines why the basic principles that underlie this book work. He hones in on the delicate balance of volume, intensity, and specificity that can make anyone a better runner.

WHEN I WAS A YOUNG RUNNER IN HIGH SCHOOL AND COLLEGE, with vastly more ambition and enthusiasm than talent, I was consumed—totally consumed—by the idea of understanding how runners trained.

I had it in my mind that if I could just find the right way to train, I would have the breakout year that would take me from being the boy who struggled to break 2:00 in the half mile, to the man who was routinely below 4:00 for the mile and was constantly a threat to break the world record or capture yet another Olympic gold medal. Hey, we all have our fantasies.

I read, and reread and reread, early publications such as *Track and Field News* and *Track Technique*. I spent more money buying books about running than I did dating girls. In college, I even had the chance to run for a week with the legendary Arthur Lydiard, the man who coached New Zealanders Peter Snell and Murray Hagberg to gold medals in the 1960 Rome Olympics and 1964 Tokyo Olympics—both of them the heroes of the dreams that played in my head while doing late evening runs on the school track. Lydiard wrote *Run to the Top*, the book that described the method he'd developed which changed the basic concept of how to train for running. Poor Arthur; I never quit asking him questions during every mile we ran together.

Well, I never quite got there as a runner. I ran 2:01.8 for the 880 as a high school junior and 4:33.8 for the mile as a college sophomore. Those are good times for normal people, but not for an athlete who was consumed with trying to run better. But I had lots of fun and made many great friends from running—running is nice in that you can talk a lot during training. And I did learn a lot about the training of the champions who I was running with in my mind. I got to the point where I could run miles and miles and miles with comparatively little effort.

Although I recognized and came to terms with the fact that I violated the first rule of sports proposed by the famous Swedish physiologist Per Olaf Astrand for becoming an Olympic champion—that is, choose your grandparents carefully—I continued to spend a lot of my professional career trying to better understand how to get the most out of training. In addition to trying all sorts of different ways of training myself, I have spent significant portions of my life with some of the major training experts in the world.

I earned my Ph.D. under the supervision of Dr. Jack T. Daniels, a running coach-physiologist who *Runners World* has called "the world's best running coach." He also wrote the book you should read after you read this one, called *Daniels' Running Formula*. Jack was, for me, the perfect Ph.D. supervisor, giving me adequate time to be the "bull in the china shop" that I tend to be in the lab—making lots of mistakes. My only regret is that I never let him coach me as a runner. I would have loved to break 2:00 in the 880 or 4:30 in the mile.

I did my post-doctoral research with Dr. David Costill, who was the guru of running in the mid-1970s and early 1980s. Then, my first boss after I finished my academic training was Dr. Michael Pollock, the scientist who conducted many of the basic experimental studies that allowed the American College of Sports Medicine (ACSM) to synthesize the basic scheme for training nonathletes: twenty to forty minutes of exercise, at 60 percent to 80 percent of the heart rate reserve, performed three to five days per week.

So, much of my life has been about what is in this chapter: questing for the magic formula for getting better at running, with the least pain, and for getting to the point where you can run with the same effortless ease (albeit with a little less grace and a little less speed) as the elite runners. It's not a quixotic or elitist dream; I have seen that almost anyone can adapt to regularly performed training to the point where he or she can move with comparatively little effort over remarkably long distances.

Training for running has a rich literature. Everyone has an opinion, a certain level of personal experience, and has read about how a certain runner trained. If nothing else, you may have read one of Sally's excellent books about training. Few people in the world have a richer experience at training people, both for competition and for fitness, than Sally. There is also a rich literature on the physiological response to training. Much of this literature is well-controlled experimental, scientific literature, where responses to various permutations of training load are evaluated over the duration of training programs ranging from a few weeks to six months.

Thus, it's easy to think that there should be a reasonable formula, defended by controlled scientific studies, for how best to train for running.

Unfortunately—and with frustration for a scientist like me—we have limited knowledge about the training of real runners due to flawed studies and poor access to competitive and semicompetitive racers. Most studies are based almost entirely on observations of newbie runners without adequate control groups, or on extrapolations from experiences of elite runners. In an ideal research world, data would be collected on veteran runners who'd stick to a serious training program for six months, which is what it takes to get meaningful results. By contrast, most of the controlled training studies we have are based on six to twelve weeks, in previously sedentary individuals. It is the classic apples-and-oranges situation.

The good news, however, is that we've collected a huge volume of information about the subject over the years. So, despite the less-than-perfect studies, we can reach some conclusions . . . which I'll share with you in this chapter.

BEGINNERS: DON'T PUSH IT FOR SIX MONTHS

Exercise training can be understood in terms of what can be called the "effect and side-effect" curves **(see Figure 7.1)** or "input-output" curves. As you exercise, your body adapts. You get fitter, leaner, stronger, and faster, and your range increases. The initial adaptations to training—usually marked by increases in the maximal oxygen uptake (VO_2 max)—typically occur over a period of three to six months, according to the ACSM standard. The effect gets relatively larger and more rapid as you increase your training load (the combined effect of frequency, intensity, and time).

If beginner runners train carefully—not too hard and not too long—positive adaptations come fast during the initial three- to six-month period, while negative effects are minimal: a little muscle soreness, the occasional tight muscle, the very occasional foot or knee pain. But if beginners train too hard (i.e., with intensity over 70 percent of VO_2 max, or about 90 percent of their threshold heart rate), it can become uncomfortable enough that most of them will lose their enthusiasm and drop out of the program. And they must limit volume, because running more than three days per week or thirty minutes per session rapidly increases the frequency of orthopedic injuries.

But if they manage to get through those first six or twelve months of training, beginners usually find that they enjoy being fitter and naturally want to see if they can go faster or farther. The time is right, because the adaptations their bodies made during the first year of training now let them tolerate increases in training load. In essence, they now want to go beyond fitness to become serious runners.

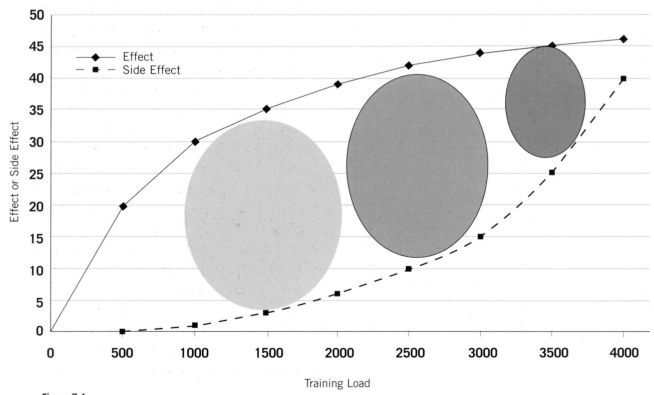

Figure 7.1

MOLECULAR BIOLOGY 101: GET STRONGER BY INCREASING VOLUME AND DISTURBING HOMEOSTASIS

Before we discuss serious running training, you must understand the training response—how the body adapts to exercise. If you skipped my Molecular Biology 101 class in college, here's a quick summary:

The interior of the cell has a certain set of conditions at rest: temperature, acidity, and the concentration of various energy metabolites. The physiology of the body is designed to maintain these conditions in a balanced way, known as homeostasis.

However, during exercise, homeostasis is disturbed. The cell gets hotter and becomes more acidic, and the concentration of energy metabolites such as adenosine triphosphate and creatine phosphate decreases. The contractile elements of the muscle also experience a certain amount of damage.

Each of these disturbances in homeostasis causes a variety of very specialized signaling molecules to come into existence. The exact details of these molecules are not important; there are hundreds of different ones, some only designed to promote the emergence of others. The key point here is that signaling molecules eventually reach the nucleus of the cell, where they stimulate some of the DNA to express itself—a fancy way of saying that the cell makes DNA copies.

Why the need for DNA copies? Well, if the signaling molecules indicate that the energy status of the muscle is very low, genes coding for the construction of new mitochondria might be expressed. If, on the other hand, the signaling molecules indicate that the contractile apparatus of the muscle has been stressed, genes coding for the construction of new contractile protein might be expressed. Thus, the nature of disturbances in homeostasis during exercise—meaning the type of training you do—causes different types of adaptations by causing different signaling molecules to be released.

But these training adaptations take time. Stimulating the construction of new proteins within the cell is a complex process that requires repeated disturbances of homeostasis over weeks and months of training. It can't happen quickly because training must be a mix of hard efforts and recovery. That means most athletes can only really train at a level to disturb homeostasis that causes adaptations two to four times per week, with the other days devoted to rest and recovery. Keeping this idea of disturbing homeostasis in mind, it's time to turn your training up a few notches.

STEPPING UP TO MORE SERIOUS RUNNING

For a certain period of time in your career as a runner, it will be enough to do your daily run, be away from other daily cares and worries, have the time to talk with your buddies and listen to music, or just feel the flow of becoming the animal you were basically designed to be. After all, beyond the scientific evidence that humans may have evolved as persistence hunters who basically ran animals until they dropped from heatstroke (Cordain, Levine), there's the simple, natural satisfaction of feeling your body respond when you attack a hill. And nothing beats hearing your spouse ask, "Are you back already?" and realizing you were running faster than normal without even realizing it.

But at some point, most of you will get the urge to "officially run"—to pay a fee, get a number to pin to your chest, have someone else time your run, and see your results printed in the small type somewhere on the Internet under the header of "Race Results." Maybe you will get a ribbon, or a little statue of a runner, or a t-shirt imprinted with "Happy Trails 10K". Congratulations—you will have entered the world of competition.

So, where is the science here? What is it that lets you go faster? Beyond the recommendation to train at a moderate intensity for about thirty minutes per day (the gospel according to the ACSM, and arguably the single best piece of health advice since someone said "an apple a day keeps the doctor away"), there is a wealth of additional detailed training data supported in the scientific literature.

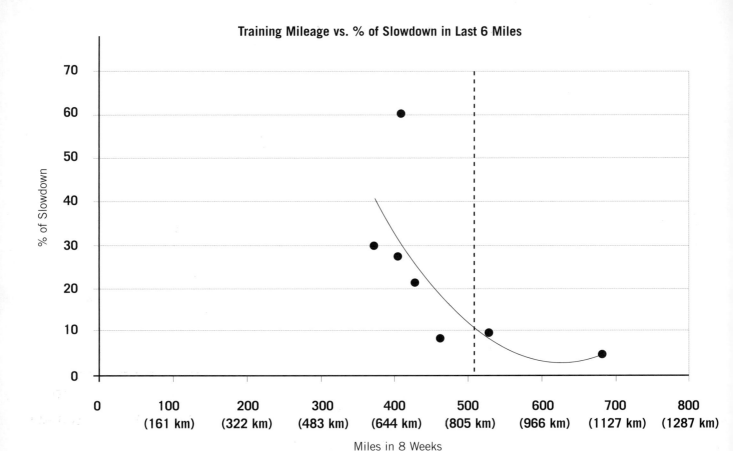

Training Mileage vs. % of Slowdown in Last 6 Miles

Miles in 8 Weeks

Figure 7.2

To make sense of all this data, we will analyze it in four ways, each covered in more depth in the following sections.

TRAINING VOLUME: THE RULE OF 3S + SLOVIC'S FOUR VARIABLES

The first thing serious runners will talk about in relation to their training is how much training they are doing. This is volume, which is typically expressed in weekly miles, kilometers, or hours.

In the mid-1970s, a statistician, named Ken Young, derived the "Rule of 3s," in which he observed that the marathon's "collapse point" (a.k.a. the wall) was at a distance that was about three times the average daily mileage performed in training for the race. Translation: If you were averaging 9 miles (14.5 km) per day, you could run three

times this far—about 27 miles (43.5 km)—before you hit the wall. That formula made the marathon, if not comfortable, then at least manageable.

The Rule of 3s was followed by a classic marathon survey report by Dr. Paul Slovic, author of *The Complete Runner*. While surveying the 541 race participants before the 1973 Trails End Marathon in Seaside, Oregon (at the time one of the largest marathons in the United States), Slovic observed that marathon performance could be predicted in terms of four variables:

- Previous mile times (which indicates general running ability)
- Eight-week total premarathon volume
- Longest premarathon run
- Number of longer runs

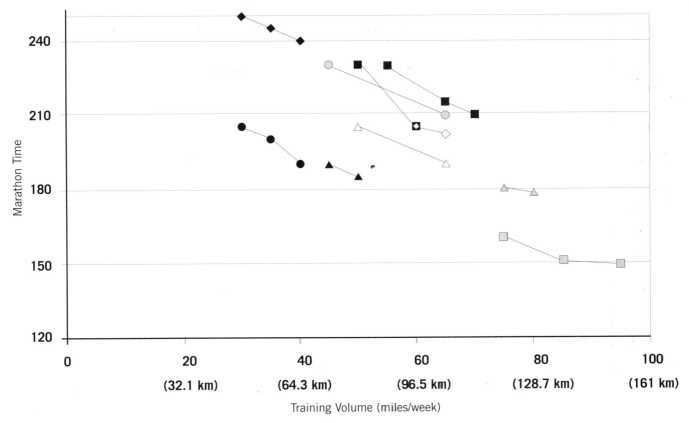

Training Volume vs. Marathon Performance

Marathon Time (y-axis): 120, 150, 180, 210, 240

Training Volume (miles/week) (x-axis): 0, 20, 40, 60, 80, 100
(32.1 km), (64.3 km), (96.5 km), (128.7 km), (161 km)

Figure 7.3

Slovic's study was published in an article titled "Distance Running" in the October 1973 issue of *Runner's World* and in the 1978 publication of his book. Dr. Jack Daniels and I repeated Slovic's study with a large number of subjects in several different marathons. Using previous running performances based on longer distances to estimate VO_2 max, we determined that our data agreed with Slovic's conclusion that marathon performance could be predicted from his four variables. We saw few abrupt slowdowns (hitting the wall) in runners who trained more than about 500 miles (805 km) in the eight weeks before a marathon, about 9 miles (14.5 km) per day and 60 miles (97 km) per week, which agrees with the Rule of 3s **(see Figure 7.2)**. Supplementing the cross-sectional observations made in survey studies, we noted improved performances over time as runners were compared to themselves over several marathons **(see Figure 7.3)**.

Achieving faster race times through increased training volume isn't just limited to marathons. My colleague Dr. Stephen Seiler, an exercise physiologist at Norway's Agdar University, found that a trend to more volume by athletes over the past twenty years is the most likely cause of improving elite-athlete performances across the board. Even in distances as short as 6.2 miles (10 km), our survey studies discovered that more volume improved performance.

Want to go even faster? Run extra-long on some days. Studies found that a very high training volume on individual days made you better than evenly distributed training. Simply put, training two hours every other day got better results than training one hour daily. The probable reason, of course, comes back to the standard run-and-rest cycle repeated throughout this book. Technically, the glycogen depletion associated with a day of high training volumes amplifies the signal to the muscle to adapt, and the off-day consolidates the adaptation.

So, again, make sure the training volume on the hard days is really hard (either through intensity, distance, or both), and the training on the easy days is really easy.

Although the Rule of 3s is a valuable guideline for training for a good marathon performance, does it apply to shorter distances, where the likelihood of a "collapse" (i.e., hitting the wall and being forced to slow down) is less likely? Logic suggests that you may need more like a Rule of 4s or 5s to do well and keep a strong pace in shorter distances. After all, if the Rule of 3s were true for 10Ks, as little as 2 miles (3.2 km) per day (14 miles [22.5 km] per week) would be ample training. Although it is true that someone who can average 2 miles per day can probably finish a 10K comfortably, it probably takes more training volume to really race a 10K without gassing out—maybe 20–25 miles (32–40 km) per week.

Figure 7.4 shows best-guess volume multipliers that a study of ours used to estimate minimal training volumes for races of difference distances. They aren't experimentally tested, but they'll give you some perspective. To run, say, 1 mile (1.6 km), you don't need to run 60 miles (96.5 km) per week to finish in good order—where you feel that you can run at your own pace and keep the pressure on. But if you don't want to start walking in a marathon, like you do when you're wasted, 60 miles (96.5 km) per week is a very good idea.

In long races such as a marathon, it's easy to forget that the final time is affected by the slowdown in the last 10K of the race as well as the pace in the early miles. An unanticipated benefit of a survey of 200+ experienced marathoners that Daniels and I did back in the 1970s as a follow-up to Slovic was that we discovered a new math-based X-Factor that could minimize the dreaded late-race slowdown: the number you get when you multiply the total

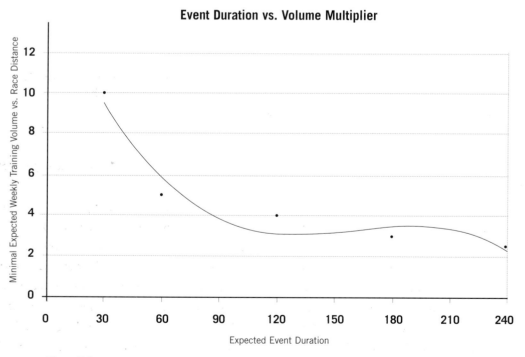

Figure 7.4

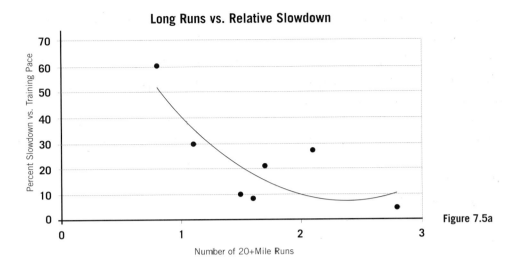

Long Runs vs. Relative Slowdown

Percent Slowdown vs. Training Pace

Number of 20+ Mile Runs

Figure 7.5a

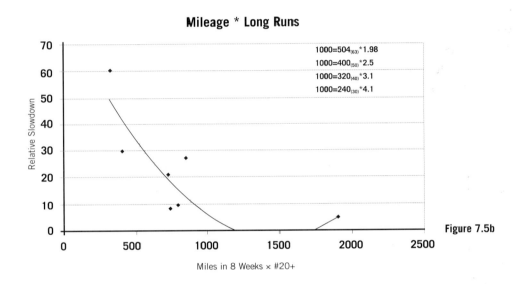

Mileage * Long Runs

Relative Slowdown

$1000 = 504_{(63)} * 1.98$
$1000 = 400_{(50)} * 2.5$
$1000 = 320_{(40)} * 3.1$
$1000 = 240_{(30)} * 4.1$

Miles in 8 Weeks × #20+

Figure 7.5b

miles run in the eight weeks before the marathon by the number of long runs in that same eight-week period. In other words, of two runners who ran the same total miles, the one who ran less often, but with more bigger-mileage days, did himself the most good.

So, if Bill and Joe, twin brothers with previously identical race and training records, each ran 500 miles (805 km) in the eight weeks before a marathon, but Bill had twenty days where he ran 15+ miles (24+ km) and Joe had only ten, Bill would be in better shape marathon day. His X-Factor score (500 × 20 = 10,000) versus Joe's (500 × 10 = 5,000) would predict that.

Bottom line: Run longer and prosper. The number of days that you go out for a run does not matter. In fact, the long runs require more rest days. We found that less-experienced runners, in particular, saw their overall marathon performance and late-race slowdown affected by the quantity and length of their longer runs **(see Figure 7.5a and 7.5b)**. It is fair to say that the longer your long training runs are, the better your results in longer races will be.

TRAINING INTENSITY

Training volume is the one thing that most runners focus on, and it indeed differentiates the very good runner from the less accomplished. But a harder training factor for runners to grasp and use regularly is one that could likewise have a tremendous impact on performance: intensity. Intensity is important because sports performance is very specific; you have to train for the sport in which you are planning to do well. Put simply, you can jog all you want, but if you want to race fast you have to train fast. At the same time, beware of too much high-intensity training. If you do too much, your performance tends to get worse, because (for reasons that are not clearly defined) your body only has a limited tolerance for high-intensity training.

This dual-edge nature of training intensity has been best articulated by, Stephen Seiler, who has noted that the training distribution pattern of serious endurance athletes in many sports can be thought of in terms of three training zones:

- Low-to-moderate intensity (in which they run in approximately 75 percent to 80 percent of their training time)
- Moderate-to-hard intensity (about 10 percent of training time)
- Hard-to-very-hard intensity (10 percent to 15 percent of training time)

These zones (which are technically defined by the blood lactate or ventilatory threshold response during incremental exercise) are slightly different from Sally's Heart Zones Training method, although they are similar in all the important ways, particularly in that they are based on intensity.

There are several basic ways to define training zones. Sally originally defined the concept in terms of percentages of the maximal heart rate (Max HR). Although that was remarkably useful, it was also a bit inconvenient in that it required measurement of a true Max HR, which probably isn't appropriate in those less well trained, particularly after they get to middle age. However, within the past decade or so, several scientists have developed methods of defining exercise training intensity.

Dr. Daniels' Training Intensities: Easy, Threshold, VO$_2$ Max, and High-Speed

My old teacher, Dr. Jack Daniels, the famed coach, physiologist, and author of *Daniels' Running Formula*, argues that there are four relevant training intensities, which he defines in terms of race or time-trial performance:

- **Easy training intensity:** A slower pace that you'd do in a two- to three-hour race, like a marathon. Unless you are planning to go for a long time, the intensity is just that: easy.
- **Threshold or T$_1$ intensity:** A race pace you'd typically keep for sixty minutes or 10 miles (16.1 km).
- **VO$_2$ max pace intensity:** A pace you'd maintain for an eight- to ten-minute race.
- **High-speed run intensity:** Essentially, these are sprints.

Daniels rotates these four intensities with various durations to optimize his training programs.

Although not grounded in the same language as the zone approach suggested by Sally and Stephen Seiler, Daniels' easy runs are compatible with training below the ventilatory threshold or lactate threshold. They are in Sally's Zones 1–4. His threshold runs are at or just above the ventilatory threshold, Sally's Zone 5a. VO$_2$ max runs are more or less in Sally's Zone 5b. The high-speed sprint runs are, well, sprint runs.

Testing Blood Lactate Response and Ventilatory Response

Identifying threshold, or T$_1$, is important because it represents the minimal pace and stress at which your body is forced to start making adaptations. Measuring it precisely is difficult, as it requires use of a lactate analyzer or other laboratory equipment. Two tests from which threshold and the other intensity zones can be accurately estimated are blood lactate response and ventilatory response:

- Blood lactate response requires a treadmill and a tech in a white lab coat who uses a special needle to prick your finger for a blood sample. The different samples, taken every few minutes as you increase your speed by 0.5 mph (1 kpmh) increments, are then analyzed for concentrations of lactate. When your levels suddenly spike higher, it indicates you reached threshold (T_1).

- Ventilatory response measures the amount of air you breathe as your running speed increases, measured by number of breaths × volume per breath. That amount increases more or less proportionately to VO_2, until you reach a middle intensity, when there is a disproportionate increase in your volume of ventilation. Part of the reason for that is you have to quickly exhale a huge increase in CO_2 and part is due to brain signals warning that extra muscle fibers are being recruited and that extra breathing would be useful.

The Talk Test: Measuring Your Ability to Talk Easily while Running

However, there are effective and faster—and free—ways to identify your T_1 on your own, without machines. The first is the talk test, the speed and corresponding heart rate at which it first becomes difficult to hold a conversation. There is an old concept that goes like this: If you can just talk comfortably when you are running, you are training at just about the right pace—it's called the comfortable talk intensity level. It's true. Don't forget it.

I remember hearing about the talk test, as it is commonly known, for the first time in the summer of 1970, from my friend Jerry Lane, with whom I ran my first marathon. We met running in the dark on the track at the University of Texas Memorial Stadium because it was too hot to run during the day. The talk test concept is much older, of course, going back to English professor and mountaineer John Grayson, who in 1939 spoke the immortal words,

"Don't climb faster than you can talk." The first systematic work on the topic was done several decades later by Toronto professor John Goode, who called it the breath-check test.

In 1998, following some early experimental work at Henry Ford Hospital in Detroit which found that talking exercisers naturally kept their heart rates within the training range recommended by the ACSM, I got together with my colleague John Porcari, the director of the Clinical Exercise Physiology program at the University of Wisconsin–La Crosse. We began doing our first of more than a dozen controlled laboratory studies on the talk test.

Our first test found that if an exerciser could comfortably recite a forty- to fifty-word paragraph during an incrementally faster exercise test (we use the "Pledge of Allegiance," but you could try anything of similar length), it meant he or she was below the intensity of the ventilatory threshold. At about the point where our runners started equivocating (finding it difficult to speak comfortably), they were almost exactly on top of the ventilatory threshold (T_1). At the point where they first declared that they "definitely couldn't speak comfortably," they were almost exactly on top of the respiratory compensation threshold (T_2).

How does this jive with Sally's system? Supervising an incremental treadmill exercise test, my graduate students Neepa Talati (2008) and Beth Jeans (2010) found that being able to talk very comfortably during sustained exercise is roughly consistent with Sally's Zone 4. At the highest stage where you can talk at all and continue to exercise, you will quickly drift into Zone 5a; few people can sustain that effort longer than forty minutes, even in a race.

How does the treadmill translate to outdoor training? You have to step down by one stage to apply it to real life. If you get a T_1 of 10 mph (16.1 kmph) on the treadmill, make it 9.5 mph (15.2 kmph) on the road. Trying to sustain a speed at which you are having difficulty speaking for forty minutes is not fun. You should be able to run at T_1 for two hours if you are very fit.

Another easy method, suggested by a study conducted by two of my 2009–2010 students, Aimee Schneider and Erica Wherry, you can do on a treadmill set at 1 percent grade (which mimics the air resistance you'd get outdoors). Starting at 4.5 mph (7.3 kmph) and progressively increasing your speed by 0.5 mph (0.8 kmph) every two minutes, you note your heart rate at each speed and keep doing this until you reach a certain point—say, 10 mph (16.1 kmph)—where you cry uncle, can't maintain the pace, and must slow down or quit. This point puts you above T_1. So, take the heart rate you had at the mph/kph just before you cried uncle—9.5 mph (15.2 kmph). This method has not been fully tested yet, but it would appear to be as good an approximation of your T_1 as the talk test.

RPE: Rating of Perceived Exertion

Another nontechnical way to estimate your workout intensity, RPE is based on your perception of your effort as you run faster, on a scale of 1 to 10. Your perceived and actual efforts may not be exactly the same, given that RPE is based on a guess. Developed in the 1970s by Sweden's Dr. Gunnar Borg, RPE tends to increase in a straightforward way as you increase your incremental speed. Although the relationship is not particularly tight, the first and second thresholds often occur at RPE values of about 4 to 5 ("somewhat hard" to "hard") and 7 to 8 ("very hard" to "very, very hard"). It is also probably fair to say that if the RPE is 2 to 3 ("easy" to "moderate"), you are at an intensity that allows you to recover (Sally's Zones 2 and 3), and if the RPE is 3 to 4 ("moderate" to "somewhat hard") you are probably in Zone 4, which is probably the place where you will do most of your training. In the RPE system, T_1 would be the beginning of RPE 5.

TRIMPS (TRAINING IMPULSE): INTERVALS, FARTLEK TRAINING, AND HEART RATE MONITORING

As we discussed earlier, training is about input and output. You do more training, you get better results. You do a lot more training; you get a lot better results. But although the formula for athletic improvement sounds simple, it is compromised and complicated by a number of roadblocks, mainly injuries and illnesses. That's why improvement is not linear as you train more; it is a decelerating curve. Bad things can increase as you train more. Here's why.

Ironically, it seems, more bad things happen to you as you train more and get fitter. The first reason is that all that hard training also makes you more tired; your fatigue can grow more rapidly than your fitness, so your performance can actually go down. On the other hand, when you reduce training before competition (the term is "tapering" or "peaking"), the fatigue fades away more rapidly than the fitness, and your performance improves rapidly. It's a balancing act.

This improvement/fatigue relationship was first described mathematically by Dr. Eric Bannister of Simon Fraser University in Canada in the late 1980s and early 1990s. The concept, one of the most complicated equations in sports, is known as TRIMPS—short for "training impulse," a way to measure the amount of training you are doing so that you can accurately gauge how your training is moving your performance ability forward. TRIMPS resembles summated Heart Zones Points, which Sally and I developed together, and therefore is central to how you think about training. But although Bannister's way is brilliant, it is rather complicated to use in practice, requiring an approach to measuring training load and input that is quite complicated.

Conveying the TRIMPS concept to you and explaining how to use it will require me to become a running historian for a few pages, so bear with me. Hopefully, by the time we return to TRIMPS, I'll have made it a little simpler than Dr. Bannister and his students did.

FIT: Frequency, Intensity, and Time

The first step to understanding TRIMPS is to understand how all training must integrate the broader FIT components of frequency, intensity, and time.

Frequency is how often you run, in days per week or month. Intensity (fast or slow) and time (long or short distance) are a little more complicated, helping you account for the hard (fast and long) and the easy (slow and short) parts of running. Your average running pace works at the simplest level, but since the effect of training to make you fitter is not strictly linear, you need a way to account for the different effects of running at different speeds.

I can clearly remember, when I was that young runner so full of fantasies of going faster, hearing other runners say something to the effect of "there's a lot of difference between running 100 miles per week and doing 100 miles of intervals." The absolute truth in this statement has led to a variety of strategies for measuring training and/or using it to define performance goals.

Intervals and Fartlek Training

Developed and refined from the 1920s through the early 1950s by German and Austrian researchers led by Helmut Reindell, Walthur Gershler, and Fanz Stampfl, intervals led to the successes of Roger Banister, the first sub-four-minute miler, and Emil Zatopek of Czechoslovakia, who gets my vote for the greatest runner of all time. (Sally might say that Joan Benoit Samuelson, who won the first Olympic marathon women's gold medal, is the greatest runner of all time.) Most often, an interval was thought of in terms of the average pace maintained for a very specific set of work/recovery repetitions. An example would be 10 × 400 meters in 63 seconds with a two-minute send-off—in other words, a twenty-minute workout that includes ten 2-minute sets each composed of a 63-second, 400-meter run followed by a 57-second recovery.

Fartlek training was also in use by the early 1950s, when Swedish researchers developed a less systematic use of hard/easy running they called "speed play" in Swedish. Not as quantitative as its German interval cousin, fartlek has you running hard (more or less at race pace) whenever you come to hills or any certain segment of road, and then continue at an easy pace during other parts of a course. The fartlek approach, like intervals, allows you to practice more distance at race pace than you could do in a single competition, and to recruit the muscle fibers that you are likely to need during competition.

For example, in a typical training day, Zatopek was rumored to have run 40 × 400 meters in less than 70 seconds each, with a 400-meter recovery jog in between. This was back in the day when running 29:00 for a 10K was a good performance. Other athletes apparently tried to duplicate this session, and virtually destroyed themselves in the process. In the early 1970s at the University of Texas, my old professor Jack Daniels used to base training around a specific interval training session, such as 10 × 400 meters with a new send-off every two minutes; the faster you run, the more rest you get. He thought that the pace you could average for the 400-meter segments was the pace you could sustain for a mile. He had runners who could average almost 60 seconds per 400 meters for the entire workout, and could almost break 4:00 for the mile. In graduate school at the time, I could average just less than 75 seconds for the workout and run 4:55 for the mile.

So, although interval training is very quantitative and systematic, and fartlek, often performed on a trail or road, rather than on a track, is less so, both are based on running segments at competition effort with recovery intervals. Both allow you a great training benefit, but also hit you with a big drawback.

The benefit: You can do high volume and high intensity at the same time, accumulating lots of total mileage at competition effort. A workout of 10 × 400 meters is 2.5 times the total distance that would exhaust me totally if I ran a mile all at one time.

The drawback: Intervals and fartlek training are so hard on your body that you can only do them a couple of times per week—maybe even just once a week—without wearing yourself down.

The solution? Run to 180 bpm, recover to 120 bpm.

Figuring out how to reduce the downside of interval/fartlek training required more information. I began to get this in the early 1970s when the interval school of thought began using heart rate as a training guide for hard/easy workouts—even though heart rate monitors weren't available yet. How was this possible? By measuring their pulse at the neck and following orders to run to 180 bpm, recover to 120 bpm.

That meant you needed to reach a heart rate of 180 bpm to create a demand hard enough to force the heart to adapt to training, and then let it drop below 120 bpm to allow enough recovery to perform subsequent efforts. The formula was convenient, too; in those pre-heart-monitor days, 180 bpm and 120 bpm also represented markers of eighteen beats and twelve beats for six seconds, which is one-tenth of a minute and an easy way to extrapolate to a full minute.

Given our current knowledge, the 180/120 scheme may seem overly simplistic. But it is worth pointing out that an exercise intensity requiring about 90 percent of the average maximal heart rate will probably lead to achieving the maximal oxygen uptake, and that a heart rate of less than 60 percent of maximal will probably not cause very large cardiovascular adaptations. If you assume that maximal heart rate is more or less 200 bpm in many young athletes, the advice to "run to 180, recover to 120" is really just advice to run to 90 percent of maximal heart rate and recover to 60 percent of maximal heart rate. This simple formula is very quantitative and effective even today, with sophisticated monitors on hand.

TRIMPS (Training Impulse) in Its Many Forms

The TRIMPS concept got rolling in the early 1990s when portable heart rate monitors that could record entire training sessions became widespread. Professor Bannister came up with the concept of using the percentage of the heart rate reserve across an entire workout as a marker of exercise intensity. Using a complex mathematical process, Bannister combined the heart rate response during a training session with the duration of the training.

TRIMPS multiplies how hard you worked by how long you worked. Does this sound like Sally Heart Zones Training System? Now you see where I'm going with this, and why her simpler way to get to the same place is such a good idea.

CLASSICAL DESCRIPTOR	CATEGORY R.
6 Rest	0
	1
11 Easy	2
13 Moderate	3
14 Sort of Hard	4
15 Hard	5
	6
17 Very Hard	7
	8
	9
20 Maximal	10

Figure 7.6

	TIME (min)	RPE	LOAD
Sunday	60	5	300
Monday	40	4	160
Tueday	70	5	350
Wednesday	40	3	120
Thursday	20	2	40
Friday	60	4	240
Saturday	60	3	180
Week TRIMP=1390			
Monotony (X/sd=1.86)			
Strain=1420 * 1.94 = 2591			

Figure 7.7a

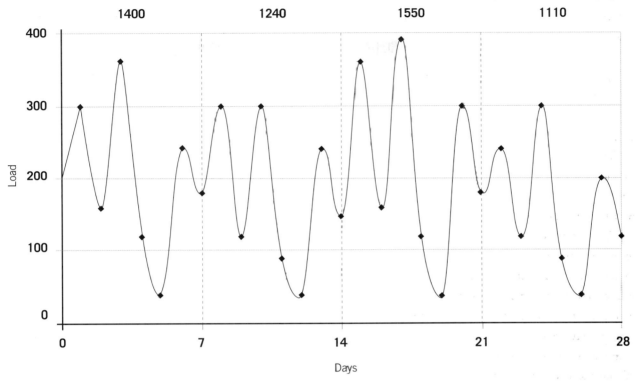

Training Load Variation

| | 1400 | 1240 | 1550 | 1110 |

Figure 7.7b

TRIMPS is an index of how much your body is provoked to adapt by training, and gives a reasonably good index of how big that day's workout was. It only needs to be integrated over a convenient period of time, such as a week, to create a training load (did you jog 100 miles [161 km] this week, or do 100 miles of intervals?). It's a tremendously brilliant concept, but very complicated to use on a day-to-day basis.

To simplify the TRIMPS approach, I went into my lab in the mid-1990s and developed what I call the Session Rating of Perceived Exertion, which piggybacks on the RPE concept discussed earlier. Instead of using a complex system based on the heart rate response, the Session RPE multiplies the RPE (your perception of the ease or difficulty of the entire workout, not just a momentary intensity marker) by the duration of exercise—thirty minutes, forty-five minutes,

and so on. The result is a number that represents the combination of training intensity and duration. **Figures 7.6 and 7.7** show an example of this simplified weekly calculation, compared with the details of the training program.

Another modification of the TRIMPS approach is the concept of Summated Heart Rate Zones, which is a much simplified method of using heart rate data to reflect the training duration and intensity. Sally originally published the concept in her book, *The Heart Rate Monitor Book*, which showed people not only how to use the newly developed radio-telemetric heart rate monitors, but also how to interpret the data.

As you well know by now, Sally's Heart Zones Training approach is anchored in percentages of the individually determined maximal heart rate and divides training intensity into five zones **(see Figure 7.8)**. Originally designed as

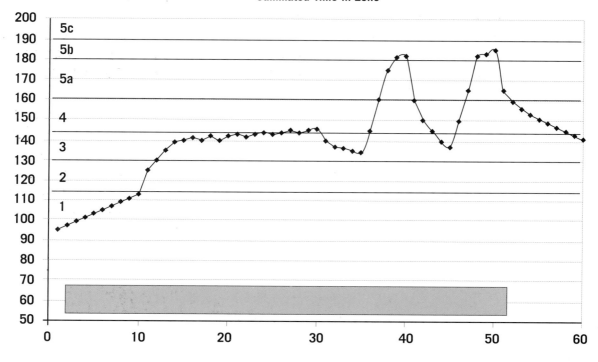

Summated Time in Zone

Figure 7.8

a system to help people characterize workouts, the system was later modified to take advantage of the download capabilities of heart rate monitors and to accumulate the time in each training zone during a workout. You calculate a TRIMPS total in the Heart Zones system for each workout by multiplying the time in each zone by the value of each zone. This is a much simpler way to get a TRIMPS than Bannister's original method.

And it does get simpler. Sally has subsequently modified her method to avoid using maximal heart rate as an anchor point, because it has problems (mainly that it may not be desirable or safe to deturmine in untrained older individuals, and that age-predicted values for maximal heart rate are so variable that they are almost worthless individually). Instead, she uses the talk test as an anchor

point, which still allows for the calculation of a TRIMPS score based on the total time in each heart zone and a multiplier for each one.

Of course, her TRIMPS score is called Heart Zones Training Points.

TRAINING ORGANIZATION: HOW HARD, HOW OFTEN

You can think of training in terms of how much total training you do (your TRIMPS score or your Heart Zones Training Points for the week) and the amount of different types of training you do during a week. The volume of training necessary is pretty well related to the Rule of 3s discussed earlier, or the volume multiplier for shorter distances. As indicated earlier, there is pretty good support in the scientific literature for this concept.

Much of what we know about training organization has been synthesized by Seiler and another colleague of mine, Dr. Jonathan Esteve-Lanao of Spain. Seiler found that high-level endurance athletes do 70 percent to 80 percent of their training in relatively low intensities that correspond to Threshold Training Zones 1–4, about 10 percent in Zones 5b and 5c, and about 10 percent in Zone 5a. He dubbed 5a a Black Hole, because at this intensity you can't go long enough to really improve endurance and you aren't going hard enough to really increase VO_2 max.

Later, Esteve-Lanao proved that to be true when he found that athletes who reduced their Black Hole time and increased their time in the easier zone improved more than athletes who did the opposite. He also found that neither group could do more than about 10 percent of their training in the high-intensity Zones 5b and 5c without burning out.

PERIODIZATION: A HARD/EASY ROUTINE THAT GETS PROGRESSIVELY HARDER OVER TIME

Almost all contemporary coaches agree that training should be periodized; there should be built-in hard days/easy days and hard weeks/easy weeks; and that training should be progressive, getting more severe (longer and/or harder) over time. This basically means the TRIMPS/Heart Zones Training Points accumulated over successive weeks should grow **(see Figure 7.9)**.

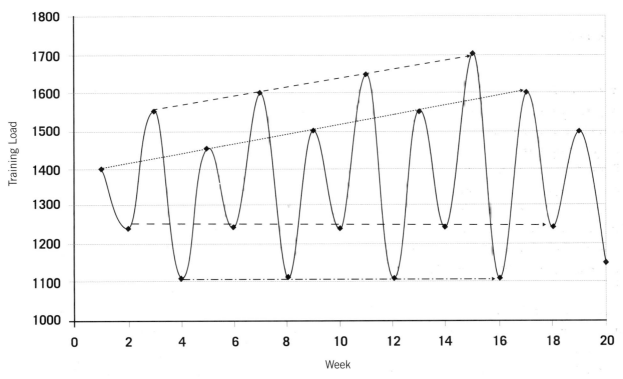

Progession of Training

Figure 7.9

It's worth emphasizing once again the cardinal principle here: Easy times are designed to be easy and to let you recover so that you can do the hard work. Everyone I know, including Sally, has such a strong work ethic that they get squeamish about the easy days or the easy weeks, which tend to feel too much like wasting time. But if you want to develop your ability to do high-end exercise—rather than just being good at training—you have to be prepared to rest when it is time to rest.

Periodization schedules can vary in different ways, and have different lengths. **Figure 7.10** presents four examples, as four-week cycles or as three-week cycles. The former is more common, as humans do seem to have a built-in four-week cycle, but the trend seems to be toward three-week cycles. In one case, the week immediately after the rest week is presented as the biggest week in the cycle (often referred to as a shock microcycle), while the other weeks during the cycle have their own rhythm, such as a bigger one in the middle of two more moderate ones.

Which periodization scheme is the best? We may never have definitive evidence. Despite lots of support for the concept of periodization in the literature, it is just impossible to adequately test the number of training permutations that coaches design, particularly for people serious enough to want a coach. Are you going to volunteer to be randomized to the control group?

Above everything else, remember that the ease of the easy days should be matched by the difficulty of the hard days. Lots of well-controlled data indicate that endurance really responds when the big days of training are really big. That's because the depletion of muscle glycogen seems to amplify the signal the trained muscles send out to turn on the adaptive process.

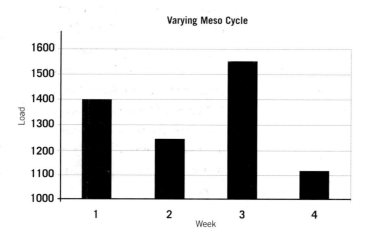

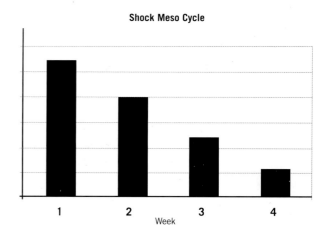

Figure 7.10

THE RISKS OF OVERTRAINING, TRAINING MONOTONY, AND TRAINING STRAIN

Some years ago, as part of a decade-long interest in the over-training syndrome (where you lose your zoom, yet nothing is objectively wrong with you), a Dutch veterinarian named Gerrit Bruin, along with a physiologist friend of mine, Harm Kuipers, conducted an experimental study of training trotters, horses that race pulling the jockey in a little buggy behind them. Race horses are notoriously easy to overtrain, and often develop a syndrome known as "being off their feed." They perform poorly, eat reluctantly, kick their stalls, and bite their handlers.

Using a hard-day/easy-day approach, Bruin and Kuipers progressively made the hard days harder, while keeping the easy days easy. They had a very large treadmill, and could run the horses until they failed. Performance progressed in the normal, decelerating-improvement fashion that one expects during training.

When the researchers could not make the hard days any harder, they made the easy days harder. The result? The horses' performance immediately deteriorated. I found this concept so interesting that I developed a mathematical way to express the amount of day-to-day variation in the train-ing load, which I called training monotony.

This term refers not to boredom, but to the degree to which your training is mono-tonic, as in "pretty hard every single day." To get technical, if you look at the TRIMPS within a week, and divide the mean load by the standard deviation, you will get an index that increases as the train-ing load becomes more similar on a day-to-day basis.
(Refer to Figures 7.6 and 7.7.)

Later, we followed up this measure of training monot-ony with another index, training strain (which is Training Load × Training Monotony). To understand how they tie together, remember that you get better as the training load goes up, but you get ill or injured as training strain goes up; since you have to have a high load to improve, the only way to control strain is to have a low training monotony.

Studying a group of speedskaters, we found that one aspect of not adapting to training correctly—getting minor illnesses—seemed to follow more or less immediately after spikes in training strain. This seemed to almost always occur when the athlete (or the coach) decided to train through planned recovery days, "just this once."

TRAINING PLAN EXECUTION: STICK WITH THE PLAN OR SUFFER

One of the most interesting observations about training that we have made is how poorly athletes execute the train-ing plan designed by coaches. I was always amazed at the amount of overtraining syndrome I saw in elite athletes—the very best human protoplasm, coached by the very best coaches. It's like a healthy person going to the Mayo Clinic for a checkup, and dying; it just doesn't make any sense.

This anomaly was focused for me by speedskating coach Stan Klotkowski, who guided the U.S. speedskaters in the build-up before the 1992 Olympics. One day, Stan had planned an easy forty-minute recovery run. To make sure the day was easy, Stan and I (two age fifty+ decidedly ex-athletes) were going to run with the skaters. Zoom! They all disappeared in front of us.

The next day, the athletes were complaining about how tired they were and how much they needed a day off. Stan, his English reflecting his upbringing in Poland, said, "If you makes recovery when I gives recovery, you not want days off."

His words were profound. Back in the laboratory, we followed the training of a group of runners over several weeks. When we independently asked the coaches what their training plan was for the athletes, we found that the athletes almost always worked too hard on their easy day. Then, because they weren't adequately rested, the athletes couldn't really go as hard as the coach wanted on their hard days. Effectively, the athletes were getting really good at training, but probably not so good at racing.

I've conducted the same experiment several other times (with swimmers, speedskaters, and basketball players), and it always comes out the same: Athletes are afraid of resting. That means they are unwilling to do what they need to do to prepare for hard training. They lose because they are emotionally lazy.

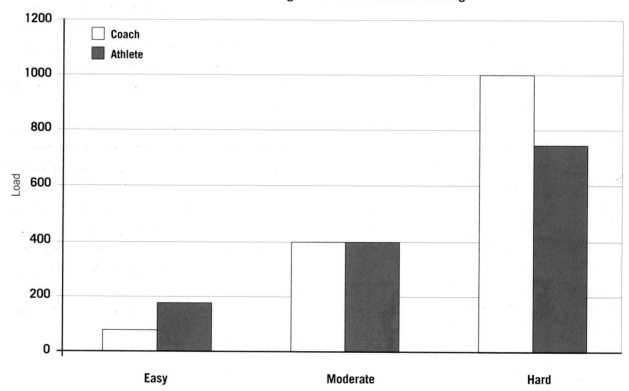

Figure 7.11

CROSS-TRAINING: USE IT TO BUILD GENERAL FITNESS AND REAL RECOVERY DAYS

One of the themes of this book is that you can use cross-training as a tool to help improve your running. Cross-training emerged in the early 1980s, first articulated by Sally in her numerous works on triathlon training, suggesting that the common cardiovascular effects of many aerobic exercise activities led to a generalized increase in fitness, regardless of the lack of muscular specificity that is usually believed to be essential to the training effect. Several studies have been conducted that used cross-training to augment running performance. Although they have uniformly been done with subcompetitive runners, they demonstrate the potential for using cross-training to improve performance.

In the first study, researchers from California State University at Northridge added cycling to the training of runners, compared to adding more running training. In these low-level runners, the performance improvement was almost as much in the combined training group as in those doing only-running training.

In a similar study done in my laboratory, we took several mid-level competitive runners and asked them to reduce and stabilize their training at thirty minutes of running, at a moderate intensity, five days per week, for approximately eight weeks. We then had them run a 2-mile (3.2 km) time trial. After the time trial, we randomly assigned them to: a) continue the baseline level of running; b) increase their running training by adding three interval workouts per week to their baseline training; or c) continue their baseline running training and add three swimming workouts per week to give the approximate total training load as the enhanced running group.

After eight weeks, everyone repeated the 2-mile (3.2 km) time trial. The results: The enhanced-running group improved by twenty-six seconds, the cross-training group improved by thirteen seconds, and the control group improved by five seconds. If you combine the results of our research with the results from the University of California–Northridge study, it appears that cross-training that is muscularly similar, such as cycling, is about 50 percent as effective as the same increase in training load performed in a specific way (running). Training that is muscularly dissimilar, such as swimming, is about 25 percent as effective as the same increase in running load.

Sometimes you can't increase the specific training load too much for orthopedic reasons, so cross-training is an attractive way to increase the total energy expenditure. As Sally's experience in her Olympic trials marathon attests, background training that is dominantly cross-training is very effective at increasing general fitness, which can then be refined by increasing specific training in the eight weeks or so before competition.

Given the strong and clear evidence for hard training days and easy training days, my feeling is that cross-training is a perfect way to do the thirty- to forty-minute duration, low-intensity (Zones 1–3) training that you do on the three to four days per week that are designed for recovery. You get low-intensity, short-duration training, and you get a break orthopedically. Then, on the three to four days per week that you plan to do hard training, you can do running training, and be recovered enough to really work on progressing the volume or intensity of the specific training.

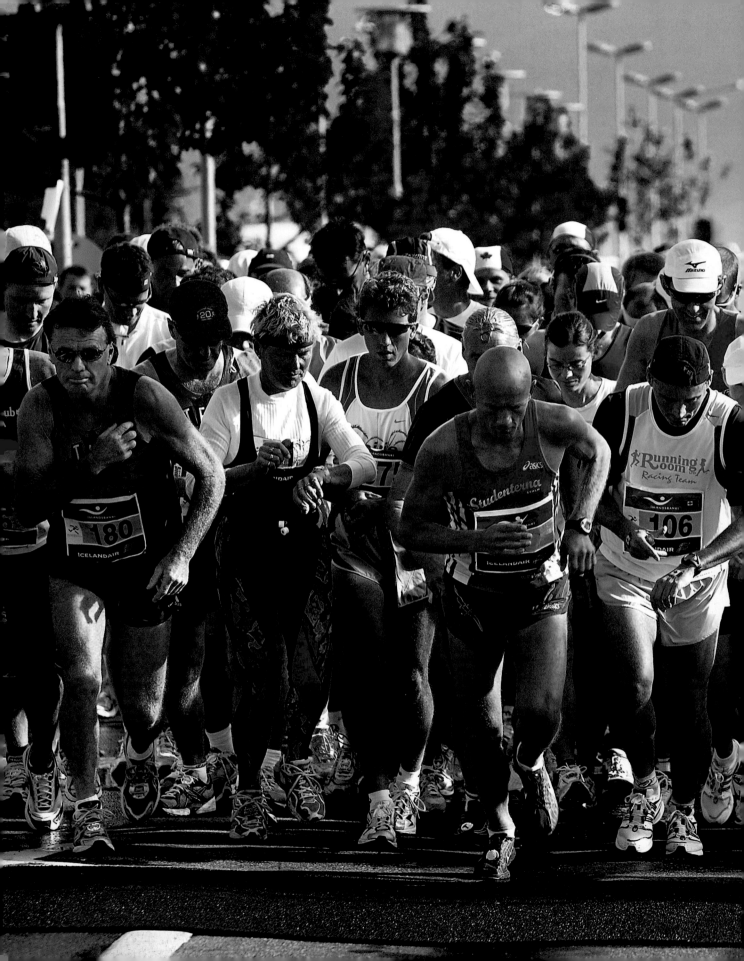

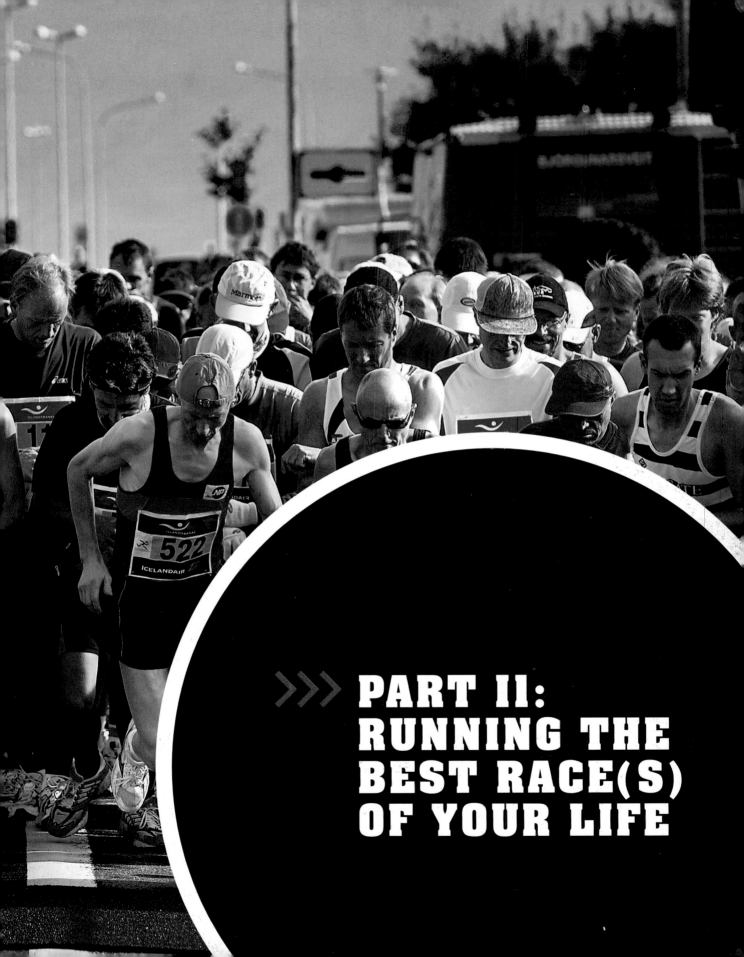

>>> **PART II:
RUNNING THE
BEST RACE(S)
OF YOUR LIFE**

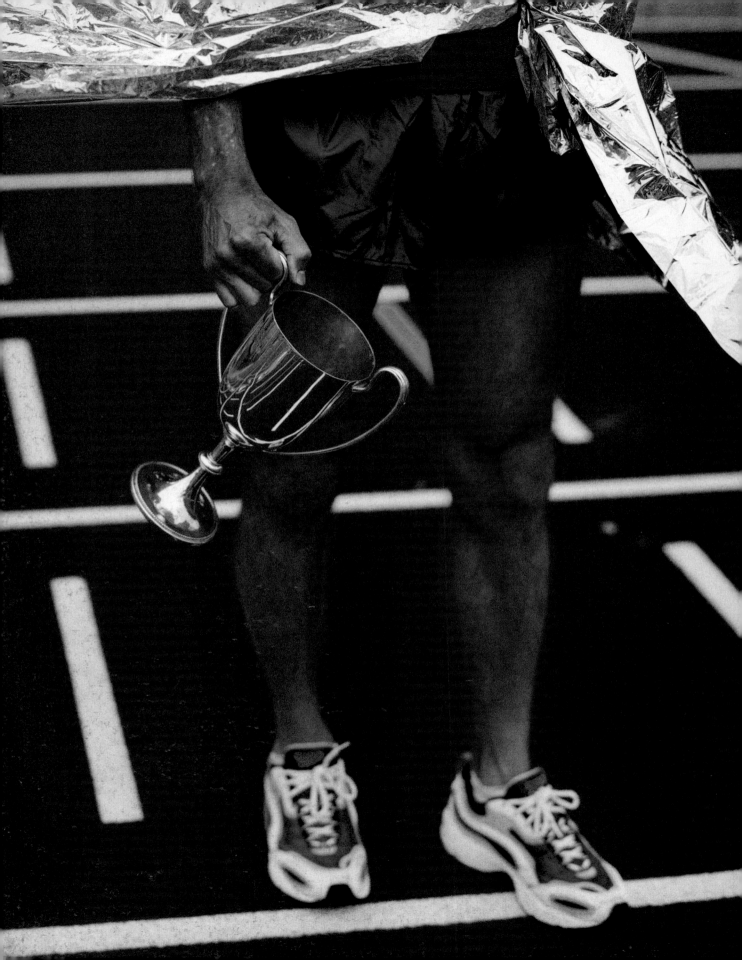

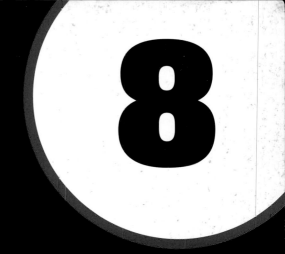

8

>>> # THE SECRETS OF SETTING GOALS: MAXIMUM MOTIVATION FOR YOUR BEST RACE

GOALS ARE THE KEY TO YOUR TRAINING They are one of the greatest gifts you can give yourself in running and in life. Here's how to establish them in the most logical, realistic, and motivating way.

MAKING IT EASIER WITH GOALS

I envy people who just get up, without a reason why, and run. For these lucky runners, no overt motivation—a PR, weight loss, general health, and so on—is necessary; somehow, running has just become such a regular, clockwork-like element in their lives that it's now simply a habitual must-do, a beyond-question routine, one of life's daily, automatic chores, like brushing your teeth or combing your hair.

I envy these people because, as much as I love running, I'm just not like that. To really enjoy running, to look forward to it and stay motivated, I need to have a fire lit under me, a reason to lace up my shoes, a real purpose for pounding the pavement or the trails. And I bet I'm not alone in this regard. I bet that most of runners out there are more like me than the guy cruising on his blissful left-right-left-right auto-pilot. Most of us need something important: a goal.

A goal gives you a reason to get out of your chair, gives your workouts purpose, and makes you chase achievements you once may have thought were beyond your reach. A goal can transform a bunch of disconnected running sessions into an around-the-world, decades-long adventure. Studies show that the very act of setting and pursuing a goal will improve your running performance and improve your life.

Because goals are so essential to enjoying running, you have to get serious about the science of goal setting. Yes, I said "science." Setting goals is a fun and valuable process that requires not only big dreams, but also a careful, realistic, even scientific analysis of what it takes to achieve them.

When President Kennedy in 1961 told Americans that the United States would put a man on the moon within the decade, he wasn't just expressing a crazy pie-in-the-sky dream that would sound impressive in his inauguration speech; he'd spoken with NASA scientists to see what was realistically possible given the country's resources, infrastructure, and potential technological progress. In the same way, you will learn to set your goals based on the talents, limitations, and potential of your own body, resources, and time constraints.

SEVEN PRINCIPLES TO GOAL SETTING

I believe there are seven principles to goal setting that you must follow to make your running successful.

MAKE YOUR GOAL CHALLENGING BUT DOABLE

Set too high a goal and you will crash and burn. Set too low a goal and you'll get bored. To get the most benefit from running for your body and your mind, don't tell yourself you need to run a 4:30 mile or a twenty-nine-minute 10K. You need a challenging but realistic goal.

ATTACH BEFORE AND AFTER NUMBERS TO YOUR GOAL

There is no greater motivation to you as a runner and athlete than seeing progress, but you must know where you started and how far you have to go—and ultimately how far you have come. Before you start your running program, weigh yourself, and measure your waist, thigh, upper arm, resting heart rate, blood pressure, even cholesterol level, and write these figures down. Then write down where you want to be in three, six, nine, and twelve months. Do not alter these numbers unless it appears clear that dedicated training leads to significantly greater or lesser results.

STAY AWAY FROM VAGUE, NONMEASURABLE RUNNING GOALS

Keep your goals hard numbers, because you can't argue with those—unlike murky, eye-of-the-beholder goals such as "feel better about myself," "have a better social life," and "make my family proud of me." All those things will happen if you meet or exceed your numbers.

BE PATIENT

If you are new to training, be aware that your body needs time to adapt. Training will be new, fatiguing, and sometimes even painful for your body. Don't risk injury; an early injury can force newbies to give up training altogether. Many coaches say to baby yourself for at least the first month of new training.

IF YOU'RE EXPERIENCED, PUSH IT WHEN YOUR BODY IS READY

Keep in mind that the large leaps in improvement that occur for newcomers are not sustainable, as they come on top of a very low base, and that if veterans still want to improve, they have to kick it up a notch. The fitter that you are when the program starts, the less you will improve in absolute terms. Don't be afraid of fartlek and interval training, at least once or twice per week; veteran runners have proven these methods effective.

AIM FOR SEVERAL MUTUALLY SUPPORTIVE LONG-TERM AND SHORT-TERM GOALS

Internal goals support external goals. Short-term goals (such as running in 5K or 10K races) support long-terms goals (such as running a marathon or half-marathon). They also give you a good gauge of how your performance is progressing.

- **Long-term running goals:** Year, multiyear, or life-long commitments that might range from nonspecific goals such as "I want to exercise four days a week with my friends and have fun" to specific accomplishments and ultimate running dreams—such as running a marathon in under 4:30 before you turn forty-five, running fifty marathons by age fifty, running a 10K in less than forty-five minutes, running the New York City Marathon in four hours, and qualifying for next year's Boston Marathon.

- **Short-term running goals:** Thirty- to ninety-day goals, often in sequence, that build you up to your long-term goal like stairsteps: a 5K in March, a 10K in April, a faster 10K in May, a half-marathon in June, a faster half in August. Each event builds you up for the next step, providing you with relentless motivation and excitement as you progress.

DIFFERENTIATE BETWEEN EXTERNAL AND INTERNAL GOALS

Internal goals are intrinsic, from-the-heart, how-you-feel-about-yourself goals. Do you need more challenge in your life? More achievement? Are you looking for more meaning? A more well-rounded lifestyle? Is there an inner you that hasn't yet been expressed, like an inner athlete or an inner child? Is there unfinished athletic business in your life? You have to ask yourself what kind of running, what distance events, what running achievements will help you satisfy your internal goals.

External goals, on the other hand, are visually focused, aesthetic objectives such as attaining a beautiful body, getting flat abs, and losing weight. These surface-oriented goals can provide powerful initial motivation, but they come with a caveat: They often don't have the depth to withstand the test of time. Surface imagery is inherently weak motivation, subject to whimsy and temptation.

THE SIMPLEST, MOST IMPORTANT GOAL HELPER: WRITE IT DOWN

The first and most important step involved in setting and achieving all the aforementioned goals does not involve lacing up your shoes or even leaving your house: Just grab a pencil and a piece of paper. Doing so forces you to focus and give real thought to what is important for your running career and your life.

Although writing down my running, triathlon, and general fitness goals is nothing new for me, given that I have been writing business plans for my various enterprises since my twenties, I know it will be odd for most people. But get over it. It may take an hour or it may take a week, and you will certainly alter it over time as your fitness and life circumstances change, but giving your goals concrete form with clarity and detail on a page makes them real. Those words, from your heart and your mind, will act like a forced truth-telling that can drive you to do your best training today and years from today. Give some real thought to the goals you write down. Then get SMART.

SMART means Specific, Measurable, Attainable, Realistic, and Timely. Those adjectives, laid out on the left side of the chart on page 123, give you a way to analyze and shape your goals so that they become appropriate for you and you alone—not for your friends and training partners.

I like to think of it in terms of greyhounds and St. Bernards. These two distinctly different breeds are each great at different things; if you are one, you simply can't be the other. If you were born with the genes, body type, and abilities of a St. Bernard, you are capable of carrying heavy loads, but you can't keep up with a built-for-speed greyhound. So, to stay happy and healthy, you must appropriately set up your goals and expectations—to beat other St. Bernards.

We set up the following twenty-section chart to help you slice and dice your goals to meet your ability—four columns listed across the top labeled "Short-Term Goals," "Long-Term Goals," "Internal Goals," and "External Goals," and five rows comprising the aforementioned SMART qualities. We filled in the chart with sample information to give you an idea of how it works:

Strategically, how your goal setting might play out over a season could go something like this: You have been running 5K and 10K races for years, by haven't been feeling much improvement. You decide that it is time to challenge yourself and set a long-term, nine-month goal of running a half-marathon while using the Heart Zones Training System. So, you scan the back pages of *Competitor* magazine for the list of races and find a local half-marathon on May 15, giving you eight months to train. You decide that a successful race experience will be measured by the following: having fun, not bonking, and meeting new people. To support this goal, you set several short-term goals, including running a 10K on March 23 and training five to six days per week using your heart rate monitor to measure improvements in your threshold heart rate.

Every day, you record your training in your appointment book with a red pen, to distinguish it from the business entries you've listed in black. You dutifully note your times and how you felt—good, bad, strong, weak, healthy, sick, injured. Following basic periodization principles, you taper for your races as planned. When you score your PR at the 10K, it's no surprise; your training log showed you getting faster. Similarly with the half-marathon a few months later, you didn't bonk and you had plenty of energy left to socialize when it was over. Mission accomplished with no surprises, all because you wrote everything down.

FINAL STEP: THE GRAND NIGHT-BEFORE RACING PLAN

When I turned fifty in 1999, I set one BHAG goal—that's a big, hairy, audacious goal, thanks to my friend Jim Collins, who coined this term in 1996 in his article on building a company's vision. My goal was quite big: Win the Grand Master division at the Ironman in Hawaii. It was hairy, too, as I would be racing to beat the best in the world in my very tough fifty-to-fifty-four age division. It was audacious— daring myself to get better as I got older.

Yep, it was a heavy, deeply personal, but worse, egotistical goal. But since I had set the Masters Ironman-distance record of ten hours and forty-two minutes at age forty (a record smashed in subsequent years), I was curious. Now, at age fifty, could I win again?

Well, I trained for that Ironman BHAG goal, and yes, I disappointed myself by finishing in about twelve hours— thirty minutes back of the winner. Although a podium finish, it was a big letdown: fourth place.

I missed my goal for a number of reasons, including that I simply lost focus on my long-term goal, letting my ego get in the way. This is a common problem with those who have trained and raced for decades. It truly didn't make any sense, in the months before, to race with an all-out effort in a four-day adventure race in China, followed four weeks later by Team RAAM, a four-woman relay team in Race Across America, a 3,100-mile (5,000 km) bike race in Southern California across the United States and ending on the shores of the Atlantic Ocean in Georgia. Sure, we won in seven days, but it just beat me up to do both of those races so close to my big goal: first place on the podium at the Ironman.

More than the damage to my body, perhaps, was the sheer distraction of these two ultra-events. If you are shooting for a win at the Big Kahuna in Kona, you better be focused. I wasn't.

So, I took my lickins and just kept on focusing and digging deeper into my serious training system for the next year. I set another BHAG outcome goal: Return to Kona and win. I told myself that this goal was daring, key, and stridently worthwhile.

SMART GOALS	SHORT-TERM GOALS	LONG-TERM GOALS	INTERNAL GOALS	EXTERNAL GOALS
S: Specific	PR in a 10-mile (16.1 km) run.	Within two years, complete a full marathon.	Feel better about myself and my emotional well-being by reducing the stress caused by not enough running. Get on a regular running program to raise my energy and improve my self-esteem within the next thirty days.	Achieve a healthy glow, which is having more energy, sleeping better, and eating smarter so that I look better and my clothes fit better in the next 180 days.
M: Measurable	• Finish in the top 50 percent of the field and break eighty minutes using both a heart rate monitor and a speed and distance GPS monitor to monitor my results. • Keep a training log and progressively increase my training load.	Improve my time by using the 10-mile (16.1 km) run as my benchmark and working to take one to two minutes per year off this year's results.	Have a complete health check (because I haven't had one in three years) and ask my doctor to provide me with the results of key tests that I want to know about. Start a record of vital physical and biochemical information on my health and fitness.	Drop one clothing size in the next six months.
A: Attainable (Action Plan)	• Write my own training plan and test it out to see if I can apply the Heart Zones Training System. • Write a racing plan before the 10-mile (16.1 km) race and preview the entire race the day before I run it. • Join the local running club and support them while I meet running partners who run my pace and effort.	• Take a VO$_2$ metabolic test to measure my aerobic fitness levels every six months.	I feel tired too much and I think that is caused by too much stress, so increase my running volume or HZT Points and take an emotional fitness test to see what my baseline stress levels are.	If my stress level is not reduced, along with my blood pressure and a few other biometrics, get professional help and support from a lifestyle coach or running coach or a specialist.
R: Realistic	Requires a commitment of five to eight hours per week of running that I must find the time for; perhaps restrict myself to less screen time.	Become fully engaged with running and change it from a hobby to a lifestyle, as this is the only way in which running will work for me. Make it a habit so that I no longer have to argue with myself whether I am going to work out or not each day.	Though I have a poor track record for reducing my workload, I know I need to work a forty-hour week to feel good about my relationships and myself. I believe that I can accomplish these goals because they are moving in the direction that I am focusing toward.	Drop one clothing size in the next six months.
T: Timely	Fill out the entry blank to an event in the next month and complete the 10-miler (16.1 km) in the next 120 days.	By January 1, have a deep base in running and be fit enough to enter 10K any day of the week.	I have tried a lot of weight-loss programs and none have worked except running. Staying on a consistent running program and eating at home rather than out is a big part of that success.	Fit nicely into my maid-of-honor dress at my cousin's wedding in April.

To accomplish the goal of returning and winning in Kona, I knew I had to make changes, changes in everything that would make me fitter and faster. I planned to cut back on my professional work hours from fifty to twenty hours per week. I bought a new, top-of-the-line $5,000 bike. I lost 10 pounds (4.5 kg) of body weight (yes, I had a little extra). I stopped drinking wine (darn). I went from vegetarian to vegan. I followed my long-term and short-term plans to the letter, just like a scientist, an applied exercise scientist that I am, would.

Then, the night before the race, I sat down for two hours and wrote another plan—a racing plan. I can hear some of you groan: More writing?

Many people say they like to take time to mentally visualize their races. They see their perfect strides, they see themselves taking the lead, they see themselves breaking the tape and thrusting their arms skyward in a giant V for victory.

Well, writing it down only makes that visualization stronger, forcing you to focus on the event in a very specific way—sport by sport, hour by hour, even mile by mile. Ultimately, it leaves you incredibly relaxed and confident, which is why I usually don't have any trouble sleeping well the night before a big race. After all, what is there to worry about when you know how the movie is going to turn out? I like to think of it as videotaping the race in your mind before it happens so that you can plug in the script as you are running it the next day.

Being a dedicated technophile, an information-based athlete, I make sure my racing plan includes heart rate, cadence, distance, and power meter data. The more data that I have downloaded into my racing plan, the better I do—and I don't think I'm unique in that way. Having your plan burned into your brain neurologically and visually by the act of thinking and writing and then reading gives you confidence, because it takes away surprise and doubt. It puts you in exhilarating control of your destiny and pushes you inexorably toward your potential, closer and closer to that peak fitness and reaching the starting line at the top of the training cycle.

The key to writing a great race plan is establishing benchmarks—for split times, for beats per minute of heart rate, for energy-sparing diet, for the perfect pace, for how much you're sweating, even for the inevitable aches and pains and the twinges that precede them. Anything and everything you can imagine or dream of goes into the racing plan.

I went to bed the night before the 2000 Ironman knowing exactly how I should feel when that starting gun fired—and thinking "This is going to be the best day of your life because you, Sally, are an athlete."

So, how'd it all play out on Ironman race day?

During the race, Leslie Sims McDowell, a strong biker who won the year before, started with an immense thirty-one-minute lead at the start of the 26.2-mile (42 km) marathon. I was seventh off the bike and certainly didn't want to be that far back at the start of the long run. But my race plan had called for me to finish the bike in about that position, and I believed that, as an elite runner, I could make up a minute a mile on her.

There's only one problem with that math: It doesn't add up to a minute a mile. Twenty-six miles (42 km) and thirty-one minutes doesn't leave me winning.

Unfortunately, the math was correct. I needed a 31-mile (50 km) marathon, and they just don't come in that distance. My nemesis won by five minutes, and I took second place.

Did I feel bad? Well, I'm a competitor, and I like to win, but this time I felt good. First of all, losing was a great motivation for the next year (which unfortunately never came, as I broke my back in a sledding accident, and soon got the degenerative disc disease that allows my vertebrae to grind on one another and prevents me from running long distances without pain). But most important that day in Kona, I did everything right. I had a clear and focused goal, I made and executed a Heart Zones Training season-long plan to meet that goal, and I wrote a racing plan that was the best that I could do that day. I raced the clock and beat the clock, but another woman simply did it faster.

After having done everything right in training, I did everything right in the race. So, I felt great and had no lingering what ifs. I was completely satisfied that I had done my absolute best. And I knew that because it was all there in my written long-term and short-term plans, my training diary, and my racing plan.

Here's the proof: In Hawaii that year, I set a benchmark of one hour fifteen minutes for swim—and got out of the water in 1:17. I was ecstatic, because one rule of the plan is what I call (based on the event) marathon math or triathlon trigonometry: Set your mark a little bit higher, just to push yourself. This is particularly applicable to the swim portion of a triathlon, given that it accounts for only about 12 percent of your total race time. So, you can really push it in the water.

You don't just pick your benchmarks out of nowhere, by the way. For the 112-mile (180 km) bike portion of that Ironman, I targeted a 150 to 155 bpm heart rate, about 83 percent to 85 percent of my max, and just 5 bpm below my threshold, with a total ride time of 6:15. These numbers were no surprise, as they were exactly in line with those I'd achieved in my training.

REFUELING AND BODY SCANNING

Of course, a thorough plan also includes more dimensions than numerical performance benchmarks. A race as long as Ironman or the marathon requires drinking and eating at regular intervals. My experience had taught me that I needed to refuel in the Hawaiian heat and direct exposure about every fifteen minutes, minimum.

And that's not all. In an all-day event, there's far more to body maintenance than diet. In fact, I find myself body scanning every three to five minutes, monitoring my thirst, hunger, sweat rate, breathing, pain thresholds, biomechanics, general energy levels, you name it. It's your body, and if you pay attention, you learn to know what it needs. If I find myself craving potato chips, I know I'm low on electrolytes. If I want a peanut butter and jelly sandwich, I know I need more sugar.

After the 2.4-mile (3.9 km) swim, I got on the bike, put my head down, checked all my benchmarks and biomarkers, kept myself fueled, and rode a steady 17–18 mph (27–29 kmph). I finished the ride in about 6:15—which was close to what I had written in my racing plan and was on-schedule given some tough headwinds that day.

On the run, my racing plan called for running at 88 percent of max, or at my threshold heart rate—172 bpm. (There were no speed and distance monitors back then, so I had to calculate my pace in my head.) I wanted to avoid the inevitable heart rate drift (the slowly rising heart rate caused by dehydration) and avoid hyponatremia (caused by drinking too many fluids), so I followed the plan and alternated water and electrolyte drinks at aid stations. I wanted even splits, set a goal of a four-hour marathon, and ended up finishing in 4:05.

Bottom line: I met all my goals that day in Hawaii. I hadn't been conservative—you can't be if you want to win. I had pushed myself to my limits and, doing the math, assumed that it would be enough for victory. I did not count on an otherworldly bike ride by my nemesis from all of these years, but I had no control over that. If everything works out, you will maintain control over your own physiology and hope that your opponents don't control theirs.

Many times, they don't. At Ironman Australia one year, I found myself ninety minutes behind the leader off the bike. It looked hopeless, but I didn't panic; I didn't suddenly push it because I knew I couldn't match that performance without blowing up. Through experience, I knew that I had no choice but to simply do as well as possible within the physiological limits I'd laid out in my plan. A few hours later, I passed that woman on the run. It turns out her killer bike ride wrecked her, and she bonked and started walking halfway through the marathon. I don't know if the plan I designed and created, the one I wrote the night before, won the race for me. But I think it's possible that a lack of a plan lost it for her.

The lesson here? Believe in yourself—and believe in your plan. Write it down, get it deep into your head, execute it, and you'll cross the line with a tremendous feeling of satisfaction no matter where you finish.

Why? Because you are the creator, you are the master designer, you are the artist of your running; it is you who sets, works for, and at the end of the event, either meets or misses the goal waiting for you at the finish line. After all, what else can you ask for? Exceeding your goal? That's an unexpected surprise that happens only when you've done your work—and the stars align.

AN EXAMPLE: BOB CROWLEY AT THE WESTERN STATES 100

Bob Crowley knows a thing or two about goals. As a principal in a Boston-area private equity firm that invests in later-stage (not start-up) companies and owns a variety of consumer and technology companies including the Vermont Teddy Bear gift company and Scribe Software, he deals with sophisticated business planning and goal setting every day. former 240-pound (109 kg) high school football player and

wrestler who didn't slim down to his current 170 pounds (77 kg) until he discovered trail running in his early thirties and has since finished more than forty ultra-running races (those over 50K), he's well versed in setting athletic goals and achieving them. But in 2010, at age fifty-three, Crowley knew he had to take his goal-setting prowess to a new level if he wanted to finish the only ultra he'd ever failed at: the legendary Western States 100, the original—and many say one of the hardest—100-mile (161 km) endurance race in the United States.

In fact, Crowley has failed to win the coveted finisher's belt buckle (silver for under twenty-four hours, bronze for under thirty) at Western States three times. He stopped on the forbidding Sierra Nevada route, which features 43,000 feet (5,486 m) of climbing and steep downhills and extreme heat and even some snow, at mile 40 (km 64) in 1994 (due to hyponatremia), mile 62 (km 100) in 1996 (due to a prerace foot injury), and mile 50 (km 80) in 2009.

"I failed in 2009 due to injuries, altitude, equipment, nutrition, you name it," he says. "I lost my confidence, too. So, to overcome both the physical and mental part of it, I knew I would have to use everything I've learned over the years."

From the start, running has always been a lesson in good planning for Crowley. "Sally Edwards was a big part of that," he says. "I met her in 1992 after her brother and I did the Ride and Tie World Championships. I'd just won a lottery slot in Western States, and since she had won the race in 1980, I asked her to help train me. She convinced me to use these new things called heart rate monitors. I quickly got faster and stronger by taking that coaching advice."

Crowley told a training partner about heart rate monitors. Although his friend ended up running his PR or personal record in Western States, Crowley dropped out less than halfway through. But he didn't let his first failure get him down, going on to set PR after PR in numerous ultras. His failure at the 1996 Western States, coupled with a commitment to his wife to help raise his young kids, did bring about a decade-long retirement from ultra-running after he finished the Vermont 100 in 1997.

In 2007, Crowley came back to the trails a different person. "I call it Tale of the Two Bodies," he says. "The first one was a young-man's body with a 3:05 marathon PR and no pain. The second one is a slower, old-man's body that is wracked with constant pain and injuries—lower back, Achilles, every possible muscle."

That old-man's body was not helped at Western States in 2009 by too-small shoes that blistered his altitude-swollen toes within 10 miles (16 km) of the start, and an anything-goes no-plan diet that had his stomach doing flip-flops. "The race chewed me up and spit me out," he says. "By 50 miles [80 km, when he dropped out], I was nauseated, cramping, seeing double, and having delusions.

"I learned a valuable lesson that day: I needed bigger shoes, and my old-guy's body could not digest solid food and run."

Determined to come back in 2010 and get the monkey off his back, Crowley sat down and built a plan.

"The first step was to build back my confidence that I could actually do a 100-miler (161 km) with body number two," he says. "So, I called a nutritionist who recommended a liquid diet, and signed up for the Burning River 100 in Ohio a couple months later—and finished it!"

Now in the right place mentally, Crowley concentrated on building his old-man's body to withstand the brutal Western States course. His goal: make himself so strong that he could take it easy during the race. "At Burning River, I'd dropped my typical, stressful, hard-and-fast, detailed race plan. My goal was to finish and have fun."

Crowley has set up a three-phase, thirty-six-week training program. Phase 1 starts with a twelve-week building phase with weeks including four days of running, two bike trainer sessions, four days of light weightlifting, and five 20-minute core days with Roman chair crunches, 70-degree incline sit-ups, and hamstrings, triceps, and biceps exercises. The arm exercises will help stave off the fatigue of carrying two 24-ounce (710 ml) water bottles or 5 pounds (2.3 kg)—all day and all night. The hamstring work balances his downhill-overdeveloped quads.

Phase 2 calls for Crowley to increase mileage by 30 percent to build speed and strength. Key to that are back-to-back weekend workouts of two to three hours of speed-work and fast tempo marathon pace running on the trails, and a four-hour trail run with his Trail Animals Running Club or Auburn running mates on Sunday. Much of this running is done in the snow and bitter winter and early spring cold of the Boston area then later in the canyons on the Western States course.

"The goal here," he says, "is to beat myself up—so Western States can't."

Phase 3 involves ten weeks of getting race-ready with at least two 50Ks and two 50-milers (80 km), followed by two weeks of tapering and protein loading to strengthen his muscles.

"By the time I hit the Western States starting line," says Crowley, "I'll have made my body strong and taught it how to burn calories, and dialed in my equipment—including size-larger shoes to compensate for swelling. I'll have put twice as much time into preparing to run as actual running—lifting, yoga, and cross-training.

"During the race, I'll ingest only carbs, electrolytes, proteins, and sodium in powder form, asking for water at the aid stations to mix my own drinks. I'll be so worry-free and in tune with my body that I'll naturally be in constant communication with myself, taking inventory from head to toe, calmly checking my body, like an airline captain on auto-pilot glancing at his dials.

"I've checked and double-checked everything that can go wrong. I've never been this prepared before."

Crowley is so serious about success in 2010 that he's permanently moving back to the Sacramento, California, area, where he got into trail running in the 1990s. "If I can make it to mile 78, where you grab that rope and walk across the freezing-cold north fork of the American River, I'm home," he says. "Literally it's my home turf, because I've run on that part of the course hundreds of times—just never in the race."

It turns out that all that preparation, learning from past mistakes, and planning paid off for Crowley. He successfully completed the 2010 edition of the Western States 100 Mile Endurance Run in twenty-five hours and forty-nine minutes, finally conquering the one race that had been his sixteen-year nemesis. "This year I ran within myself, checking my heart rate monitor constantly to make sure I wasn't going out too fast. My fueling plan of drinking 85 percent of my calories (~300 calories per hour consumed) and having the opportunity to train in the canyons on the actual course made all the difference. I gained valuable confidence and insight that enabled me to just relax on race day and enjoy the journey home." And enjoy he did, looking strong aid station after aid station and through the night. "My personal struggle to complete this journey over two decades has made the finish all that more satisfying. I feel humbled, blissful, and cleansed."

CREATING YOUR PERSONAL MISSION STATEMENT

If you are struggling with the concept of goal selection as it relates to running and athletics, it may be helpful to start with a broader perspective of your life to identify your ultimate motivation. A mission statement is a short, all-encompassing, self-description commonly used by companies to define their purpose as a producer of goods and services, as an employer, and even as a corporate citizen with impact on the community, nation, and world. I have found it useful in setting a foundation for myself and my various personal and business enterprises. You may likewise find it a useful base from which to branch out to goals in running and other aspects of your life.

To give you an idea of the challenging, satisfying, and fun process of creating and refining a mission statement, which will certainly change over the years as you do, here's a page from a diary of mine that describes a mission-building moment in the summer of 2009.

"This summer I struck out on my annual birthday-celebration backpacking trip with my two hiking partners, both of whom are Seattle marine biologists. The first hiking partner travels with the trail name Hi-Fi-Di (she's a high-fidelity gal) and the second with the trail name Aye-Aye-Aye (one of the most positive women I know). My chosen trail name is The Head Heart.

We began our ten-day, 125-mile (201 km) adventure on the Pacific Crest Trail excited to be away from our daily lives. Our long-term goal is to hike the 2,600-mile (4,184 km) Pacific Crest Trail from Mexico to Canada by hiking it 125 miles (201 km) each summer, for however many summers it requires.

On day four, Hi-Fi-Di opened the conversation and shared that she couldn't figure out the next step in her life. She said that she is dissatisfied and frustrated with her home life, her work, and her relationships. Looking for answers, she asked us, her dear and trusted friends, "I thought I'd be further ahead in life than where I am now—and it's my forty-eighth birthday?" That is one bodacious question. How many people think they should be further along than where they are finding themselves as they head toward the halfway point in life: age fifty?

I suggested that we use the Hippocratic method of asking questions rather than giving opinions or solutions to try to solve Hi-Fi-Di's question. Hi-Fi-Di was suffering from a loss of direction and a frustration with her current life's location. After a full day of our questioning Hi-Fi-Di as we hiked through nature and mountains, she was able to come to a definition of her life's problem. That was our first step. The next day and the next step, Hi-Fi-Di brainstormed twenty-five strategic actions. We helped her prioritize the strategies by selecting which would most help her accomplish her life's mission. Then, she whittled the list down to five strategies that she believed she could successfully accomplish in the next year.

That's when it came together that she couldn't do it alone. Hi-Fi-Di proposed that we form a personal board of directors, a P-BOD, to support her. And as we ticked off 10–15 miles (16.1–24.1 km) per day of rugged trail hiking, finishing each day swimming in a mountain lake, eating a hot dinner under billions of stars, and falling asleep happy in our sleeping bags, we repeated the process. In turn, we each spent a day sharing our issue, defining it, creating a mission description, making a list of strategies and whittling them down to what could be accomplished, and signing up to be members of each other's P-BOD. We signed up to be there for each other.

The result is that now we have a support system and accountability plan with our new P-BOD. We have each written our personal life statements and shared them with each other—and I posted mine in my office so that I read it everyday. We have agreed to support each other by checking in quarterly, and to hold a P-BOD meeting to assess quarterly progress. The official annual meeting is next summer as we again hike another 125-mile (201 km) segment of the Pacific Crest Trail. It is our plan to be each other's support system and P-BOD members for the next twenty years (although it probably will take us a bit longer than that to complete 2,600 miles [4,184 km]).

I thought I'd share the final mission statement that I created with my P-BOD during the hike through Northern California's Sierra Nevadas. After six decades of living and given my current location and direction, the mission statement is as follows:

PERSONAL MISSION STATEMENT—Sally Edwards, Sept. 2009: To be highly successful getting America moving while living a fulfilling and productive life with my loved ones.

Can I challenge you to write your own PMS and burn it into your mind and daily activities?

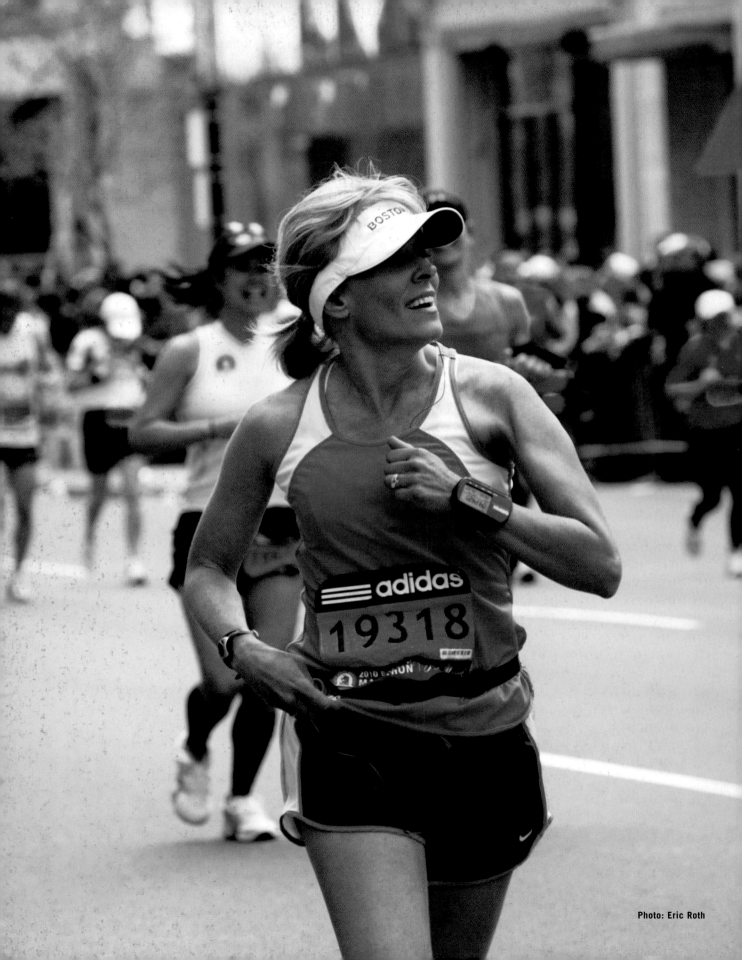

Photo: Eric Roth

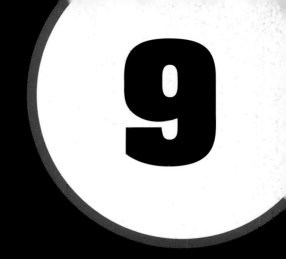

RACING AT YOUR BEST:
BEING IN TOP FORM ON RACE DAY

RACING CAN BE INTIMIDATING. After all, it's so much harder than running. Running—what we do during training—is a comfortable, fun, motivational thing, full of the excitement of improving, the camaraderie of working out with friends and sharing training stories, and the feel-good encorphins of the so-called "runners high." But then comes race day, and all those enjoyable aspects of the sport suddenly disappear. If you experience even a sliver of those warm-and-fuzzy running-training feelings during a race, according to Carl, consider yourself lucky. Because racing—real performance racing versus "just-want-to-finish" racing—is not comfy and fun, mentally or physically. In fact, physiologically speaking, he says, if you do it right, it only feels good when it's over.

Understanding that and the reasons behind it is important, because you'll realistically know what to expect during the race—and how to race it to your best. Then, after you've achieved your goal and made yourself proud, you can go home, collapse on the couch, and return to your old carefree days of just simply running. Until the next race, that is.

WHAT'S HAPPENING TO YOUR BODY DURING TRAINING

Carl has a Ph.D. and world-renowned expertise on this subject, so I'll let him explain it in his own language:

Running, and exercise in general, is about disturbing homeostasis—about changing the current conditions in which your body is fully relaxed to something a bit more stressful. Imagine a situation in which you are sitting in a comfortable chair, a couple of hours after a nice light meal, listening to your favorite music. The temperature in the room is comfortable; you don't have to sweat or shiver; you aren't repairing any injuries, and you haven't really had a hard workout in a couple of days, so there is no soreness from the last workout. Also, your last meal wasn't too long ago, so you aren't hungry, yet it wasn't too heavy, so you don't have that stuffed feeling. You are listening to nice music, so you are relaxed and carefree, with no particular worries, work problems, or family problems to solve.

This is homeostasis, the condition on the inside that your body constantly strives for. It's the condition where your physiological processes are idling at their lowest level; perhaps the most difficult thing your body is doing is breathing and circulating blood to provide just enough energy to keep your body temperature above the room temperature and replacing the few cells in your body that are ending their natural life cycle and being shed. In some ways, in homeostasis, the hardest thing your body is doing is growing your hair and your fingernails.

During your normal daily run, you disturb homeostasis. You are using energy faster than at rest, so you have to continuously replace the chemical adenosine triphosphate (ATP) in your muscles, which is the energy source of muscle contraction. Because humans are not very efficient animals, your running metabolism is only about 20 percent efficient (meaning that about 80 percent of energy we produce is heat; in cycling, the efficiency is a bit better, about 25 percent, and in running it is less efficient).

The upshot is that as a runner you will accumulate some extra heat, the biggest single waste product of metabolism, so you'll be sweating lightly, enough so that your body temperature is only slightly above the 98.6°F (37°C) that is typical at rest. To provide the extra energy for the run, you are breathing harder, and your heart is pumping harder (both at a higher heart rate and at more blood per beat—at i.e., a higher cardiac output) than at rest.

But so far, all of these physiologic responses are within the limits of your body to cool itself. Providing the energy for running and for keeping conditions near enough to their homeostatic norm just isn't very hard. If you are used to exercising regularly, it actually feels pretty good. Although the science behind the so-called runner's high is far from perfectly clear, most regular exercisers report a rather pleasant feeling.

WHAT'S HAPPENING TO YOUR BODY WHILE IN A RACE

When you race, however, you are working close enough to the limit of your ability to maintain homeostasis, so conditions on the inside of your body progressively deteriorate.

In response to the disturbance in homeostasis, your body responds more and more aggressively to it in ways that are easy to recognize. These may be less than perfectly pleasant. You are breathing harder, your heart beats faster and faster, you get hotter and hotter on the inside. That usually means you sweat more and more, your muscles sense the disturbances in homeostasis and send signals to your brain, which, in effect, say, "What are you doing to me? Why don't you slow down? It would feel a lot better if you did." You know what happens next: The brain doesn't listen.

You have some silly idea in your head that it would be good to run a mile in four minutes, or 10 km in 40 minutes, or a marathon in less than three hours, so your brain ignores the signals. In the process of ignoring the signals, and pressing on with your racing pace, the signals get stronger and stronger. Eventually, the signals your body is sending out to your body will win, and you will slow down.

If you slow down just as you cross the finish line, you are probably pretty happy with the result. If, however, you have to slow down before you get to the finish line, you are probably less happy with the feeling, and are definitely less happy with the result.

As for the distance of your race, it's a given that the nature of the disturbances in homeostasis are quite different depending on the type and intensity of muscular activity you attempt. Your body will not feel the same and your mental struggle to overcome your body's protest will be very different during a 5K than during a marathon. The 5K is about heavy breathing and burning legs; the marathon is about "winding down," or "wearing out," and it just goes on for such a long time.

Carl's final advice is Viva la difference! Race a lot of distances, and enjoy the way your body and mind experience different races. Some of you are built for the long endurance races and some of you are built for the shorter, faster races. Try them both. Discover what you are genetically built for and race a lot to learn.

SALLY'S RACE DAY DOS AND DON'TS

After three decades of racing at the front and now at the back of the pack (I volunteer to serve as the official final finisher at races so that no one else gets saddled with that distinction), I see both sides of the racing experience. As a result, I know the dos and the don'ts of racing about as well as anyone.

DO WARM UP

- **It's essential.** Consider the warm-up part of your race. Don't start any race cold. Jog, do some sprints, stretch some. Don't do enough to get fatigued.
- **Show signs.** Have your heart rate slightly elevated with a little sweat on your forehead and under your arms as you toe the starting line, which are physiological indicators that you are warmed up and ready to run hard.

DO KEEP THE PACE

- **Start slow.** For races longer than 5K, start out a wee bit slower than you think you should, and finish faster. This is the 49 to 51 percent racing rule: Run the first half of the race at 49 percent of your projected finish time, so you can finish the second half at 51 percent. The slow start is important for a long race because it allows for a gradual warm-up, helps you avoid the hare-and-the-turtle phenomenon, and keeps you strong for the last half, leaving you plenty of gas to push it harder to the end.
- **Take it to the limit.** By the end of the race, if your goal is to do your best, you should be exhausted—with nothing left in the tank.
- **Cool it in the sun.** In the heat, expect a slower finish time. Start more conservatively than usual, drink more along the way, and, if you need to, take a cue from the much-respected Olympian and author Jeff Galloway, and walk occasionally. He says that if your goal is a five-hour marathon, you could even program in a one-minute walk every six minutes; for a six-hour marathon, a one-minute walk every four minutes.
- **Take the tech advantage.** Strap on your training tools and use them, even if it is a simple sports watch with time splits. Start using data, beats per minute, minutes per mile, temperature, average heart rate, and other information to keep you on the beat and on the mark.

DON'T TRY NEW GEAR AND BIG MILES

- **Use time-tested gear.** Don't try new shoes, new foods, new clothing, or a new running pace on race day. You don't want to work the bugs out on game day.
- **Beware the big leaps.** Don't do a marathon as your first race. There'll be too many new things coming at you to learn on the fly. Work up from a 10K, and half-marathon—and take good mental notes of everything your body is feeling.

DO DRESS FOR SUCCESS

- **Wear white.** Dress in white apparel with UV protection to stay cool. Some fabrics will reflect the sun when wet.
- **Use your head.** Wear a hat to prevent sunburn and glare.
- **Tight might be right.** Consider bicycle-style shorts (without a pad) if you have a history of crotch chafing.
- **Love the Lycra.** Avoid cotton socks, which can cause blisters. Lycra socks designed for running hug your skin and protect better.
- **Consider "run-way" fashion.** Wear flattering running clothes that will motivate you to run confidently.

DO EAT

- **Wake up and chew.** For all race distances, you need energy, so eat breakfast about two hours before a race, waking up earlier than normal if necessary to allow digestion time and gastric emptying.
- **Top off the tank.** If you feel the need no less than thirty minutes before the race, eat half an energy bar, half a bagel, a banana, or a high-calorie/low-acid food for an extra energy boost.
- **Listen to your body in the long run.** In-race eating is a very individual thing. Ideally, you will have already experimented with nutrition during training runs to find what works best for you. Usually, during a long run or after a workout, your body will tell you what it wants— peanut butter, energy drink, banana. For most people, nutrition does not become an issue until distances longer than 10K, usually starting with a ten-miler (16 km) or a half-marathon.
- **Enjoy the sixty-minute scarf-down.** On long races eat something every hour—whether you feel like it or not.
- **Partake in a finish line feeding frenzy.** To aid recovery and feel better that night, immediately eat and drink when you cross the finish line. The forty-five-minute window immediately after any run is when the body is most receptive to refueling for energy restoration.

DO HYDRATE

- **Thirst comes first.** This may sound obvious, but always drink when you are thirsty. Don't space out and forget. If you get behind the eight ball, distressed from dehydration, it is very hard for the body to process liquids fast enough to get back on track.
- **Drink more than water.** Although drinking plain water is fine for races under an hour, since you have enough fuel and electrolytes in your body to handle that, marathons require more fluids with nutrition and salts. In the second half of a long race, do whatever it takes to replace salt and electrolytes—electrolyte replacement drinks, nonacidic fruit juices, even a sprinkle of salt in a cup of water from an aid station. In the early days, I made my own replacement drink out of bee pollen, aspirin, and salt. Then I switched to Gookinade, the very first commercial energy drink on the market, because it was the first lab-tested source of fuel and electrolytes blended into powder form.
- **Count to fifteen.** Drink at least every fifteen minutes. To prevent liquid from sloshing around in your stomach, it's better to drink a little bit (about 1 oz, or 30 ml) frequently than a lot all at once.
- **Every hour, drink a pint or two.** Depending your size and sweat loss rate, drink a water bottle's worth—14–27 oz (414–798 ml)—per hour.

DON'T OVERHEAT

- **Help the core chill out with water and ice.** Do all you can to keep your core body temperature low. The body must release internal heat, which will hinder the function of vital organs. It does this and cools you down by kicking in your natural thermoregulator, which shunts the blood supply away from the stomach, intestines, and bowel and to the skin for temperature regulation, bringing blood to the skin, where it cools off next to the ambient air. You can aid the process with water and ice, frequently splashing the surface area over large, blood-carrying arteries in your neck; washing your entire face (which, if overheated, wrecks your mood and performance), and snagging some ice at an aid station and putting it in a scarf around your neck, in your hat on top of your head, or elsewhere.

- **Stay hydrated.** Keep in mind that blood supply to working muscles and vital organs drops as blood pushes to the surface, so don't forget to drink 1 oz (30 ml) or more per mile (or km) to maintain blood volume and cardiac output. (For you technical types, remember that $CO = SV \times HR$, or cardiac output equals stroke volume times heart rate.)
- **Keep your feet dry.** At aid stations, pour water over your head slowly so that it doesn't drip in your lower body and shoes. If your shoes and socks get wet, it is an open invitation to blisters and sore feet.

DON'T LET YOUR BIOMECHANICS GO TO HELL

As you get tired, your running technique may crumble, which slows you in two ways: It exacerbates fatigue simply because you lose your efficiency, and it can lead to inefficient breathing. To guard against form breakdown in the last 25 percent of the race, when it is most at risk, do frequent body scanning, mentally going from your feet to your head. Check your posture, keep your chest open, keep your back tall (not straight), and run with quiet foot strikes.

DO KEEP SAFETY IN MIND

- **Lube it.** Use body lube such as Sportslick or Vaseline wherever your body parts rub, blister, and chafe, including between your toes and below your armpits.
- **Nip it.** Men may choose to apply nipple bandages or tape to prevent irritation and possible bleeding.
- **Clip it.** A week or so before the race, clip your toenails short enough to keep them from jamming the inside front of your shoes. If you have hardened calluses, consider having them shaved off to prevent blisters.

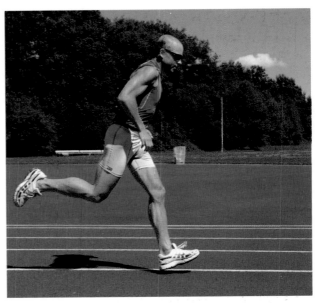

This runner shows poor form typically seen at the end of a race. His shoulders are rounded and his body is leaning into his stride; this causes his foot to strike more heavily and exacerbates his fatigue.

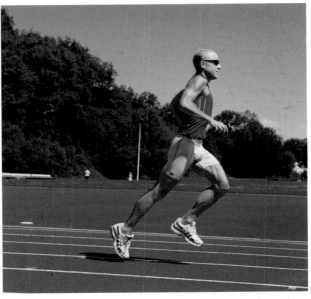

This runner has maintained proper biomechanics and running technique. His chest is open and his back is tall but not stiff. His hips are under his shoulders and his foot strikes are light.

Faido, Faido, Faido!

For years, I held the women's marathon record for the Ironman triathlon with a time of three hours and twenty minutes. The first year in which prize money was awarded to finishers, rather than trophies, that record was demolished.

While I was amassing trophies, not cash, during the sport's infancy, I decided to enter the Ironman World Series, which consisted of a points series of five Ironman races around the world, all in one year. After finishing the first three races in the series, I suffered a devastating bike crash, winding up in the hospital with a level-three separated shoulder, concussion, and major rehabilitation and loss of training time to prepare for the next Ironman.

I made it back with the fourth race in the series in Japan on a beautiful course that finished at a fifth-century castle surrounded by a moat with a bridge that led to the finish line—a baseball field.

In Japan, as I raced to a PR and a new world master's record of ten hours and forty-two minutes (which has long since been smashed), I heard the crowd along the sidelines of the marathon shouting "Faido, faido, faido!" The words send back to me huge pangs of remorse. That's because I missed my two Fidos, as I assumed the Japanese called them, who were surely waiting for my return. If you are a dog-lover like I am, you know how much you miss your canines when you travel.

But it turns out that the Japanese view of faido was not what I thought at first. One day, my mind, directing a set of marathon-running legs, latched on to an idea: I was in second place; could it be possible that faido meant that the crowd was trying to encourage me and let me know my place in the field?

After I finished the race, I asked an English-speaking Japanese race official to translate the word *faido* into English. The official explained that to the Japanese, *faido* means "to fight."

Next, I told her that I had spent a year during the U.S. war in Vietnam from 1970 to 1971, volunteering with the American Red Cross, and that my father was a war hero—the first pilot to take off during the bombardment of Pearl Harbor in 1941. (I also told her I, too, had a definition of "to fight" that was associated with fighting.) But I was wrong again.

The official said that to the Japanese, "to fight" means to fight against the voice, the power that is inside you and encouraging you to quit, to give up, to slow or to stop. And that when they yell "faido" they are encouraging runners to fight against what is inside them that keeps them from doing their best.

- **Zip it.** In a race-belt pocket, carry several essentials such as cash, some form of ID, and a telephone calling card and medical insurance information.

DO A THOROUGH PRE-RACE PREP

- **Time-trial your race pace.** Know your race pace before you get to the starting line. Time-trial half the distance at race pace ten days or so before you race. If your goal is a forty-five-minute 10K, do a 22:30 5K to test out that pace. After the time-trial workout, ask yourself whether you could hold that pace for another 5K distance in race conditions.
- **Know your heart rate.** When you do your time-trial run workouts, assess your average heart rate in the same conditions and terrain. If you perform better during races with data (as I do), knowing your heart rate ranges during the run helps enormously in terms of motivating me and keeping me on my goal pace.
- **Check out the course.** Try to train on the actual race course. If you can run the course in advance of the race, you might do better. The day of the race you will have the comfort of familiarity as well as the information on terrain, scene, and environment.

- **Avoid surprises.** Try everything before the race: apparel, gear, fluids, shoes, just everything. You should not experience any equipment or nutritional surprises during the race because you are familiar and have broken in all of your gadgets and gear in advance.
- **Make a plan with your team.** If you are going to do the race with your training partner, talk about the "what ifs" in advance. My first 100-mile (161 km) race, my training partner and I decided to stay together for the race—come hell or high water. When she overheated and chose to sit in a cold mountain creek for an hour, I stayed with her. When she dropped out of the race at mile 62, I picked up the pace, and finished third wondering what might have happened if I had decided to run it alone.

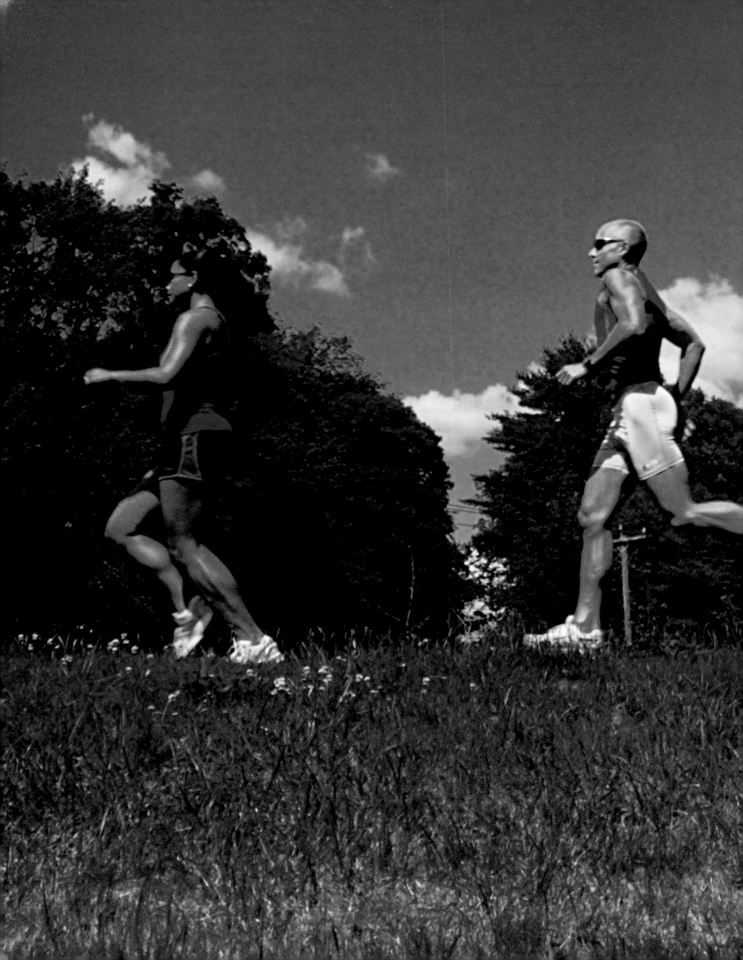

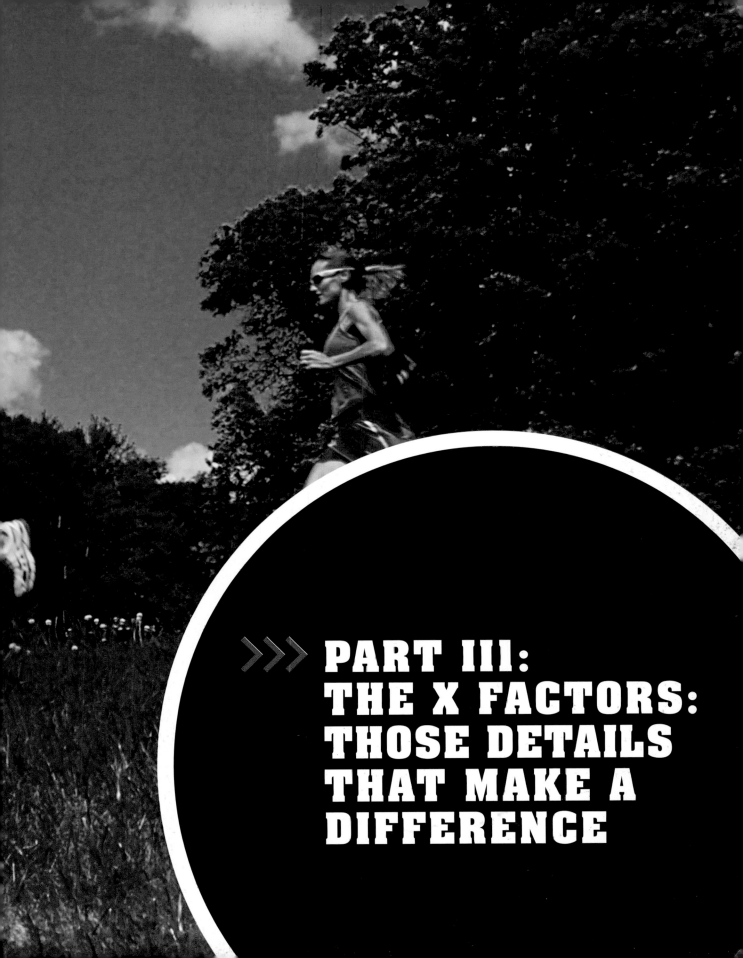

>>> **PART III:
THE X FACTORS:
THOSE DETAILS
THAT MAKE A
DIFFERENCE**

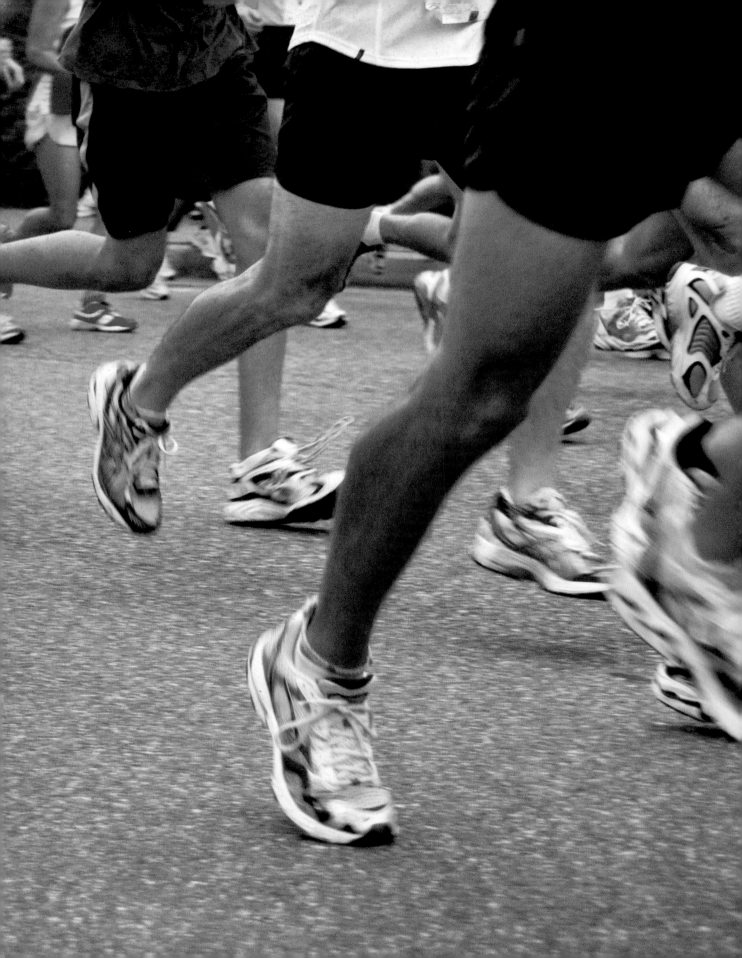

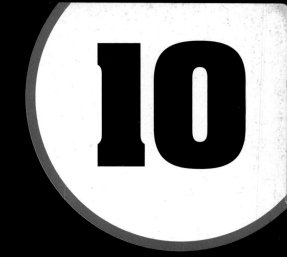

>>> FORM: FOREFOOT, MIDFOOT, REARFOOT, OR BAREFOOT?

FORM IS A TOPIC THAT HAS NEVER RECEIVED MUCH ATTENTION in the running world. For decades, few coaches and magazine columnists had much to say about it, other than "don't worry about it—run whatever way feels natural." While I have learned over the years that there are ways to make your natural form more efficient, which I'll get to in the following pages, form has none-theless stayed in the background behind three things: training, training, and more training. Long before Czechoslovakia's Emil Zatopek won the 5,000 meters, the 10,000 meters, and the marathon at the 1952 Olympics with a running style many thought that he looked like he was "a man having a heart attack," the topic of form has basically not been on the radar for runners.

That is, until the year 2009. During the writing of this book, the interest in running form skyrocketed virtually overnight. That was due to two factors: the publication of the best-seller

Well . . . I refuse to get swept up in the hysteria. Being a career-long heel striker who's seen many things come and go over the years, I view this new obsession with barefooting as a mere blip on the screen of this sport. I don't see it as sustainable for most runners. I view it as a fad that won't last long. People want to land on a soft surface, and will not give up the protection and cushioning of shoes. And they may find it causes more injuries, not fewer injuries.

As a proud early adopter of sports technology, such as heart rate monitors, I certainly have no fear of new ideas. Among those are the very cushioning technologies that Lieberman and barefooters are tarring as evil: Being in running-shoes retail for two decades, and completely immersed in the world of running for four decades, I have seen these features help too many runners and prevent injuries to suddenly agree they are the embodiment of evil. I pride myself in methodical, numerical analysis and proof. I crave facts. And the facts thus far tell me that running injuries are not caused by shoes, but by training errors, the relentless day-after-day, steady-state, repetitive-motion running that we explicitly warn against in this book.

Can barefooting help reduce injuries, as many claim, or is that an illusionary panacea, no more than wishful thinking? With the number of barefoot adherents still tiny, and common sense telling me that not many people are going to run barefoot on pavement much after they try it a few times, there are not a lot of facts to go on. So, I'm reluctant to hop on the barefoot bandwagon, and instead I issue this word of caution: We can't tell if unshod running will stop long-term injuries, nor can we tell tell whether it will cause new ones.

BARE BEWARE: BAREFOOTING CAN BE A HASSLE, WRECK YOUR RUNNING ECONOMY, AND RISK INJURY

Changing your form ain't easy. The changes that I recommended in the preceding section are relatively minor in the scope of things, but still difficult to implement. So, imagine the trouble you might have trying to incorporate more substantive changes to your form.

For an example of a substantive change, let's take belly breathing, which is breathing through your nose during aerobic activity. This type of breathing theoretically allows you to suck more oxygen down into the large bottom portion of the lungs, which is often underutilized during shallow-breath mouth breathing. I completely agree that nasal or belly breathing is a good, logical idea; accessing your whole lung, not just a fraction of it, is sure to make you perform better. The trouble has to do with practicality. I couldn't run while nasal breathing. I gave up after a few tries, and went back to my open-mouth panting. And I don't think I'm unusual, because I've never seen a marathoner breathe only through his or her nose and get on the podium.

This goes to show that it's hard to make a change even when you know it would be good for you over the long run. By the same token, years of dong things one way make it hard to adopt a form that is natural, even biologically programmed into your ancestors. Like barefoot running.

"Yes, we're predisposed to run barefoot on soft surfaces," says Carl, who occasionally ran barefoot drills on the infield as a college miler at the University of Texas. "But I don't know of anyone who doesn't get hurt running barefoot on concrete, and I just don't agree with Pose and Chi running (which promote shod barefoot-style forefoot/midfoot landings to reduce injuries). Give me a soft, springy surface to run on and I'll gladly run barefoot. But if I have to run in twenty-first-century America, give me some shoes.

"That's because everybody finds his or her own most efficient way to run," he continues. "Jack Daniels [noted running author/researcher and Carl's Ph.D. advisor] looked at forefoot and rearfoot strikers and asked them to change [to the other style]. His findings: Energy costs [the amount of oxygen required to run a certain distance] went way up." It was more "expensive" to change styles because the runners had to suffer through new, unusual biomechanics.

The bottom line? "Mother Nature is very smart," says Carl. "Something very bad happens when you try to change your form."

As I understand it, then, if you get used to doing some things the same way for years and years, even if it's technically the wrong way—like, say, my style of heel striking—your biomechanics learn to accommodate that form.

Heel striking has worked great for me. That's one reason I'm against barefooting, besides worrying about glass and thorns. Barefooting's forefoot/midfoot strike will completely mess with my natural heel-strike biomechanics.

Certainly, Barefoot Ted, Dr. Lieberman, and Christopher McDougall would instantly argue that a "natural heel strike" is an oxymoron—that the cavemen who evolved over 500,000 years of barefoot living simply couldn't heel strike. And that the only way I can is because I wear shoes with a big thick cushion on the heel. And it's true: Take your shoes off and heel strike. You can't do it; it hurts. But you must remember that we simply don't live in that environment anymore—and haven't for thousands of years.

Your barefooting form is, by definition, as personal a running form as you're going to get, but it evolved for running in grass and dirt. It did not evolve to run on concrete, which the Romans invented 2,000 years ago and, from the looks of the drawings, only walked and ran on with the protection of sandals. In the modern world, cushioned sandals protect us so much that we can heel strike, even though we tend to do it less as we speed up.

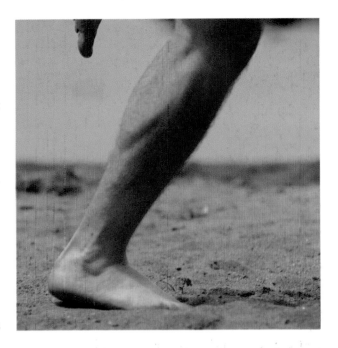

Yes, you can happily run barefoot on concrete, as Roy Wallack's report will show you, especially if you don't run into a rock or a piece of glass. However, the common Achilles and calf pain that dogs new barefooters indicates that some major biomechanical relearning must occur. Some adapt to the new landing pattern within a few weeks, and some never do. Some may not mind having to pay more attention as they run. And some may find out, as I mentioned before, that different injuries crop up over the long term. We just don't have enough data yet to know and to recommend it to you, especially if it penalizes your running economy.

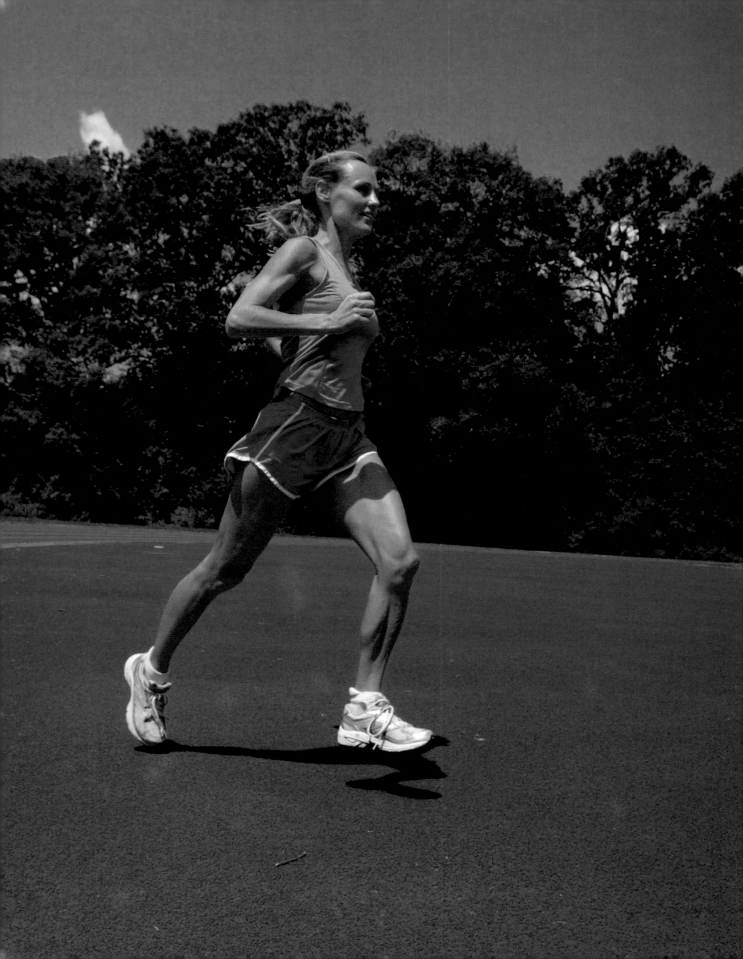

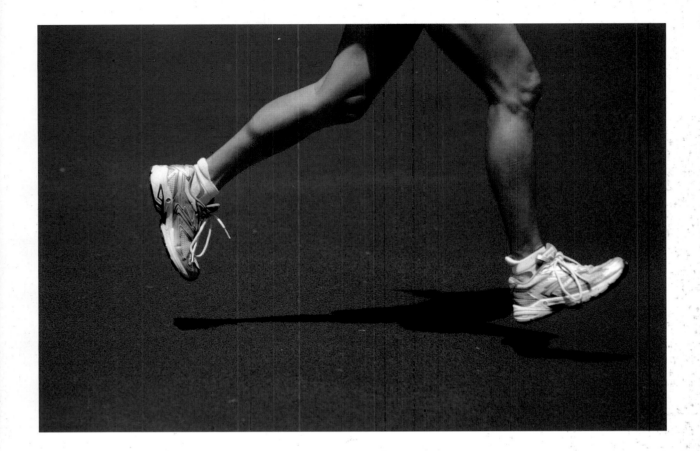

Ultimately, I think making a radical change to your established shod running form is not worth it. It's difficult, uneconomical, and an invitation to injuries. Most people won't have the patience to make the change. Besides, it might be unnecessary, as most injuries can be avoided by a hard/easy, high-zone/low-zone training regimen.

But as I have stressed again and again, running is a highly individualized endeavor. There is no ideal running form, no one-size-fits-all approach. So, for the sake of efficiency, longevity, and pure fun, you owe it to yourself to experiment.

Try different speeds, shoes with thick cushioning and no cushioning, novel training tools (such as my e3 Grips—see Chapter 11), and innovative training methodologies—even far-out ones such as barefooting. Go to clinics and use what works for you. I enjoy running with a heart rate monitor and an MP3 player, but that may not be your thing. Use yourself as your own test dummy. The more variety your feet and body experience, the more balanced and healthy you will be as a runner and athlete.

BAREFOOT TED'S NONSTARTER

Ironically, my wait-and-see attitude toward barefooting was somewhat validated by an incident I had recently with a colorful barefoot-running icon. In November 2009, I was asked to appear at a runner's forum the Thursday before the Sacramento (California) CoreLogic Cow Town Marathon, serving as the emcee at "A Night with Barefoot Ted McDonald," the barefoot runner who—along with barefoot running itself—had rocketed to fame over the previous several months as a featured character in Born to Run. More than sixty people showed up in the little Clark's Corner latte shop in the Sierra Nevada Gold Country town of Ione, some from as far as 200 miles (322 km) away. All had read the book, and were plenty intrigued, but a quick show of raised hands showed that none of them had yet run barefoot.

Barefoot Ted was sponsored for the evening by CoreLogic's founder Craig Klark, who became intrigued after reading about him in the book. He then was planning to stay the weekend and run the marathon.

Ted and I were a good contrast. He was a former chronically injured shod runner who kicked off his shoes to become a now-famous trumpeter of barefooting, a radical, new idea that he said would revolutionize running and eliminate forever the injuries that strike 60 percent of all runners per year and stunt running careers decades too early. And I was the traditionalist, a dyed-in-the-wool member of the establishment, founder of a well-known shoe-store chain, a firm believer in cushioning, control, and dual-density midsoles, and unconvinced by the sudden tsunami of interest in barefooting, which I hadn't tried myself and had dismissed as a fad.

It was Mr. Barefoot versus the Queen of Shoes.

Ironically, as I discovered, Barefoot Ted isn't purely barefoot. He spoke at length about the injury-free bliss of barefooting while wearing his signature Vibram Five Fingers, a thin-bottomed shoe-glove with individual toe compartments that is said to let you mimic barefooting, and which he sells on his website. Ted was ardent and colorful in retelling his tales from the book and describing the purported benefits of barefooting, which he said was poised to explode from its tiny band of zealots into the mainstream. He enthusiastically outlined the now-well-known argument that barefooting/Vibram-ing (no difference between the two, he said) forced you into the natural shock-absorbing form that our homo sapien ancestors developed in a million years of pre-civilization barefoot living—specifically, landing you on your forefoot, not your heel, thereby reducing shock to the knees and hips. He mentioned how his injuries evaporated entirely when he dumped the supposed sensitivity-deadening cushioning of running shoes and went exclusively to barefooting six years before, and how he'd seen his story repeated in hundreds of other barefooters.

Given his earnestness, I got a shock when I talked to Craig Klark, the organizer, a week later. "How'd Barefoot Ted do in the marathon?" I asked.

"Oh, he didn't do it," came the answer. "He was injured."

Wait a minute. Injured? Barefoot Ted, the barefoot poster boy, too injured to run a marathon a couple days after regaling an audience with barefooting's anti-injury prowess? Hmmm. I tried not to make a big deal over it, but it did put a cloud over the message that he was giving. This was like a morals-touting politician being caught in bed with a prostitute he charged off on his government-issued credit card. To his credit, he did finish the 5K run, albeit injured, in a twelve-minute-per-mile pace.

BAREFOOT MAY BENEFIT SOME RUNNERS

Not everyone agrees with me on the value of barefoot running. Roy M. Wallack, one of this book's coauthors and a *Los Angeles Times* fitness writer and columnist, runs barefoot regularly. Roy was one of the first to cover the barefoot/Pose Method scene with stories in *Runner's World*, *Men's Journal*, *Men's Fitness*, *The Los Angeles Times*, and his own book *Run for Life*. Like many runners, Roy believes that one injured day for a barefooter, even one as illustrious as Barefoot Ted, doesn't delegitimize barefooting, or mean that it doesn't have something to offer.

Here is Roy's report on barefoot running. Although unsure about the mass appeal of barefooting, Roy believes it is a worthwhile option for all runners and that it has been a lifeline to some chronically injured runners at risk of giving up the sport. Although my own experience with barefooting hasn't led me to adopt it, I think the answer to most questions in this world is "it depends," so I will pass the baton to Roy for a close-up examination of the barefoot trend. Read the next section for his unique and enlightening perspective on this new, high-profile activity of interest to many runners.

FIELD REPORT: UP CLOSE AND PERSONAL WITH THE BAREFOOT REVOLUTION

I'd ridden on the Bolsa Chica bike path in Huntington Beach, California, hundreds of times in my life. It never dawned on me that one of my biggest revelations would come from getting off my bike, taking off my shoes, and running on it.

Surprisingly, that's what I found myself doing for 3 miles (4.8 km) one sunny afternoon in February 2004. "Feels good, doesn't it?" said the forty-eight-year-old man with long hair, a long beard, and a quick wit who was running beside me. He was Ken Bob Saxton, who I would soon know as the exalted guru of all things barefoot. And he was right. It did feel good.

I discovered Ken the day before when I Googled "barefoot running," which was one of the inspirations of the Pose Method, a radical new anti-injury running method winning thousands of triathlete converts that I was writing about for *Runner's World* magazine. It turns out that Barefoot Ken Bob, as he's known, was the real deal. He had finished twelve barefoot marathons that year with a PR of 3:27 that qualified him for Boston, which he'd be running in six weeks. A computer technician at Long Beach State who been biking barefoot 12 miles (19.3 km) to work everyday, he'd given up shoes in 1987 when they gave him blisters at the Long Beach Marathon. With his relentless editorializing about the evils of shoes ("they deaden your feet, make you run imbalanced, cause injuries") on his website, Runningbarefoot.org, and growing publicity through occasional magazine and newspaper features on him, he'd become the leader of a tiny but growing barefoot movement. "Come on over and I'll teach you how to do it," he told me. The tutorial was quick: Take off your shoes.

There was no learning, per se. I followed Ken to the beach. Not to the sand, but to the bike path. I cringed, looked at my toes, and started jogging.

Then an amazing thing happened: nothing. Pounding the pavement didn't hurt a bit. In fact, it felt great—almost like a massage. My toes spread wide, as if I was gripping the path and "reading" the terrain with the bottoms of my feet. And my running form felt remarkably natural and smooth. Instead of clumping along with my normal heel striking, I automatically ran softly with short strides and a squatted form while landing on my midfoot before quickly touching the heel and lifting the foot. On top of all that, I found myself wrapped in a childlike joy that was almost addictive.

When we finished, I was speechless. Yes, I'd landed on a couple of little pebbles, as Ken warned, but my light landings minimized the momentary pain and allowed me to flick my foot up almost instantly. All in all, I felt great.

(continued on page 148)

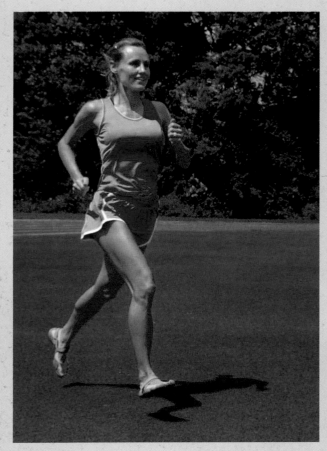

A slightly crouched posture makes your legs absorb some of the shock of running barefoot.

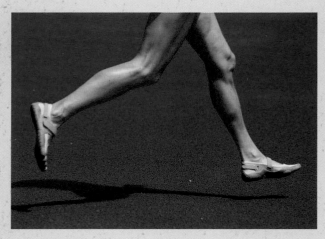

When running barefoot or wearing Vibram Five Finger shoes, land on the midfoot or the ball of the foot.

My right knee, never quite right after a torn meniscus surgery six months earlier, hadn't felt this good in a long time. Ken warned me that I'd pushed it too hard for a first timer, that my calves might hurt from the new biomechanical load (and they would, for a couple of days afterward), but it didn't matter; my eyes were wide open. Could barefoot running be more than a quirky ritual performed by a vegetarian hippy? Could it offer some real benefits to mainstream runners?

To find out, I called the Olympic Training Center (OTC) in Chula Vista, California, where I was surprised to hear running coach Todd Henson go on effusively about barefooting.

"We always warm up and cool down with barefoot running," said Henson. "It's actually become more important as shoe technology has gotten better." He soon began to sound like he was channeling Barefoot Ken. "Running shoeless can prevent injuries and improve technique," he said, "even if you only do it for a few minutes before your regular run. It works because it restores feet to their natural state, before they were stifled by shoes. Shoes do a swell job of protecting your feet from snow, rocks, and smack needles and the like, but over time they desensitize the tiny sensors in your feet that tell them how to react to their environment. Eventually, feet grow lazy and weak, triggering a chain reaction up the entire leg that can lead to shin splints, jogger's knee, and ITB strains. Big cushiony heels can just add to the problem, shortening calf muscles and the Achilles tendon. Running without shoes stretches out the calves and gets foot muscles moving again. It's like push-ups for feet."

"You see a lot of athletes with great engines but flat tires," said another OTC coach, the legendary Brooks Johnson, known for his work with Regina Jacobs, Patti Sue Plummer, and other future Olympians at Stanford University from 1979 to 1992. "Barefoot running quickly pumps back up the tires. It gets the foot back to normal."

(continued on page 150)

▶ Good barefoot running form: When running barefoot, you should be slightly crouched and your forefoot should be striking the ground immediately before your heal

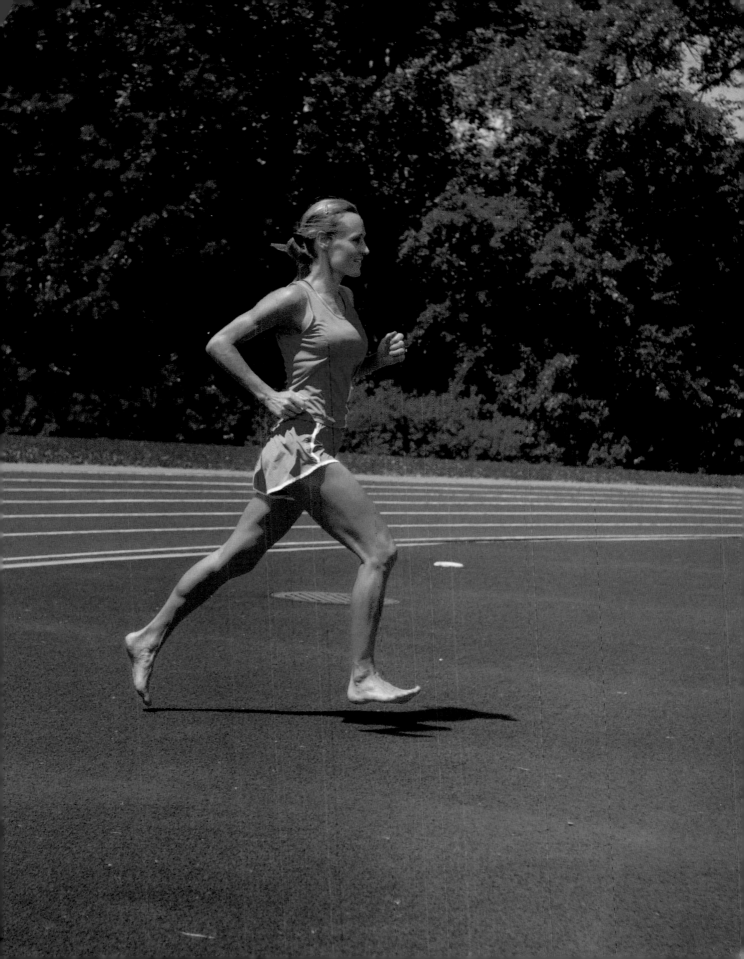

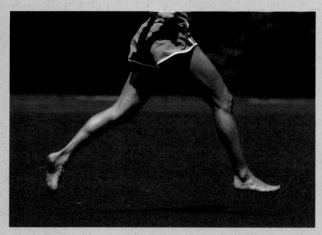

When you use proper form you land on your full relaxed foot, not the heal or the ball.

Academic researchers have also had positive things to say about the injury-prevention aspect of barefooting, which is its main draw for average runners. In 2003, a group led by esteemed South African researcher Dr. Timothy Noakes, author of the seminal, 930-page tome, Lore of Running, found that a forefoot landing can reduce shock to the knee by as much as half over that of heel strikers in cushioned running shoes. The study, "reduced eccentric loading of the knee with the Pose running method" in the March 2004 issue of the American College of Sports Medicine's (ACSM) *Medicine & Science in Sports & Exercise*, compared heel-to-toe runners (heel strikers) to a control group trained in the Pose method invented by Russian sports scientist Dr. Nicholas Romanov, who says he modeled it after barefoot running.

"I was quite surprised at the magnitude of the change," Noakes told me, noting that the reduction for nearly all the runners was "more than 30 percent—with some as high as 50 percent. We have seen nothing else that does this—not shoes, no matter how padded," he added. "I think the Pose and barefoot running is advantageous in preventing injuries, which is quite important since we know that roughly 60 percent of runners get injured every year. It is highly probable that the Pose method would translate to [fewer] injuries, although this is not conclusive since we have not studied that."

Noakes and several biomechanists I contacted, such as Keith Williams at U.C. Davis, did warn of the potential for calf and Achilles pain, given that a forefoot landing would be new for most people. Romanov himself said the calf requires a two-week strengthening period. Williams said any radical biomechanical change like this could take as long as six months. This jived with my experience and those of many Posers and barefooters I've interviewed for other barefoot-running stories over the years. Some people never get comfortable with the forefoot landing or accompanying rapid turnover and revert back to their old heel striking.

As I write this in the post-*Born to Run* era in 2010, Ken Saxton has racked up more than 100 marathons and has become a true running celebrity who appears in the pages of *Runner's World* virtually every other month, the traffic to his and other barefoot websites and running clinics has exploded, the interest in barefoot-in-shoes methods such as the Pose and Chi running has mushroomed, and the demand for "barefoot shoes" such as the Vibram FiveFingers and the Panka FeelMax is insatiable. I've interviewed average folks who turned to barefooting to cure injuries and never looked back, and others who reverted to shoes quickly. I met hardcore barefooters such as Alex Romero, a Cal Tech Ph.D. student in evolutionary biology who ran a 2:40 to win the 2009 Duke City marathon in Albuquerque, New Mexico. His brother Julian came in second at 2:47, also running barefoot. They are proof that barefooting need not slow you down, once you get used to it.

Barefooting recently drew some additional academic support from the Running Professor—Dr. Daniel Lieberman of Harvard, a featured player in the book *Born to Run* who has long argued that long-distance running was critical to human evolution and development. Seven years after Dr. Timothy Noakes' landmark finding that barefoot/Pose running cut knee shock in half, Lieberman drew similar conclusions. His study, "Foot strike patterns and collision forces in habitually barefoot versus shod runners," published in the January 2010 edition of *Nature* (and partially funded by Vibram), concluded that "fore-foot and mid-foot strike gaits may protect the feet and lower limbs from some of the impact-related injuries now experienced by a high percentage of runners." His study suggests that running barefoot or minimally shod is a more natural and healthier way to run than heel striking in traditional cushioned running shoes.

Disagreeing with some of Lieberman's findings—in particular his stamp of approval for minimally shod running—is Barefoot Ken Bob Saxton, a proud "pure" barefooter not as open-minded as his friend Barefoot Ted McDonald. "Putting anything between your feet and the ground deadens your feet and corrupts your natural form," says Ken. "You need to learn how to run barefoot before you use Vibrams, because they will allow you to run unnaturally." Posted comments on Ken's website often concur. "VFFs made me sloppy, although still better than I could have done in shoes. I just didn't have the feedback I needed to make sure my feet were landing right or picking them up right," wrote one runner. To that end, Vibrams are expressly not welcome at Barefoot Ken Bob's Saturday morning barefoot running clinics.

Bottom line: The high injury rate in running is a fact. It may come from training incorrectly (which this book addresses at length), heel striking, wearing the same shoes all the time, or, most likely, a combination of all the above. For the sake of their knees and their running careers, I think that frequently injured runners owe it to themselves to jettison the heel strike forever. (Most will find that sprinting, a method for finding your ideal form, naturally will eliminate heel striking.) As for footwear, I think you should "cross-train your feet"—alternating between barefoot running, Pose and Chi running in regular trainers, and forefoot/midfoot landings on all surfaces in minimal-shod footwear ranging from Nike Frees to racing flats to Vibrams. Like running

on road and trail, cross-training makes you stronger. Ultimately, any option is worth exploring, as long as it's different from the one that is injuring you.

THE BASICS OF BAREFOOTING CORRECTLY

1. Run crouched:

A slightly crouched, bent-knee position that sets you 2 or 3 inches (5 or 7.6 cm) below your normal erect standing height helps turn your leg into a shock-absorbing spring and sets up a soft barefoot landing.

2. Get on the ball:

Land on the forefoot/ball-of-the-foot, with the heel off the ground. This avoids the high-impact heel strike landing that leads to the injuries that cripple many runners.

3. Let the heel touch down:

The heel should be allowed to touch the ground immediately after the forefoot does. Do not try to keep the heel off the ground, as this will overload and stress the calf and Achilles tendon.

4. Flick the foot up fast:

After the heel touches down, instantly flick the entire foot straight up toward the butt, shooting for a cadence of 180+ steps per minute. The longer the foot is on the ground, barefoot or shod, the greater the chance of injury and the greater the amount of body weight that will be applied to trail and road obstacles like rocks and glass.

5. Don't do too much too fast:

Since barefooting involves a natural, but long forgotten biomechanics, you will overstress many unused muscles and connective tissue if you jump right in with your normal shod mileage. Start with 5 minutes and gradually work up to allow your body to accommodate to your new natural form; also use it as a warm-up and cool-down for regular shod running to strengthen feet and legs. Avoid the fate of many enthusiastic beginner barefooters, who often suffer injuries that force them to reluctantly return to the shoes that led to their problems in the first place.

TRAIN RIGHT: YOU'LL AVOID INJURIES AND FIND YOUR OWN FORM

Roy, Carl, and I all agree on some things. Hard day, easy day. Stress day, recovery day. And stay out of the Black Hole. This simple training philosophy, which you may remember from Chapter 3, makes you stronger by pushing hard enough on your hard day to mobilize your body to improve itself and then allowing enough easy recovery time on your recovery day to lock in the gains. And in doing so, it also limits injuries.

"The trouble is that people don't do this," says Carl. "They run too much and too many days in a 'more efficient' row at the same pace." The average runner strikes the ground with a foot about 1,000 times per mile (1.6 km)—3,000 to 5,000 times in a thirty-minute run. And because of all that impact, he says, it does not matter if you wear cushioned shoes, racing flats, or no shoes at all—you will get hurt. Repetitive motion leads to repetitive-motion injuries, period. That's because the smallest, otherwise-inconsequential biomechanical inefficiencies—and we all have them—eventually awaken from their slumber when they are repeated over and over. What you do or don't wear on your feet simply does figure into this equation.

The solution? "Go hard, go easy," says Carl, "so you're not repetitively loading the same stride. And you're giving yourself time to recuperate."

The takeaway here is that changes in your speed, running surfaces, and terrain will provide a variety that minimizes repetitive motion. The hard/easy training template is a simple, effective way to accomplish that—and will make you a faster runner, too.

The hard days also serve another function: They actually train you to get injured less by rewiring you with more efficient biomechanics. In other words, hard, fast running sessions teach you a better, safer form.

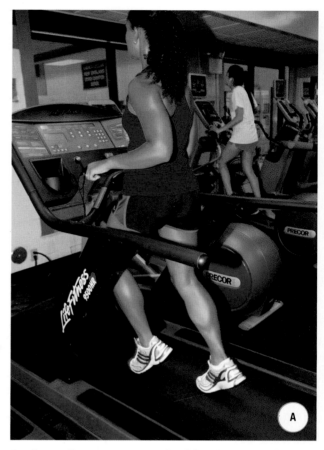

Running at a T_1 recovery pace—a slow, leisurely pace—on the treadmill. The hands are low and relaxed.

I realize that my use of the term "better form" may seem contradictory, considering that I, Carl, and 99 percent of running coaches think there is no such thing as an ideal running form. But it makes complete sense if you personalize it—that is, individualize your training and biomechanics. Here's what I mean:

Carl often sums up the debate over running form (and his opposition to attempts to change it) by saying "you are what you are," but he does not mean to imply that what you "are" is static. To borrow a phrase from the U.S. Army, you as a runner ought to "Be all that you can be." Translation: Your running form/style/ergonomics can be improved, but it won't necessarily be improved by copy-

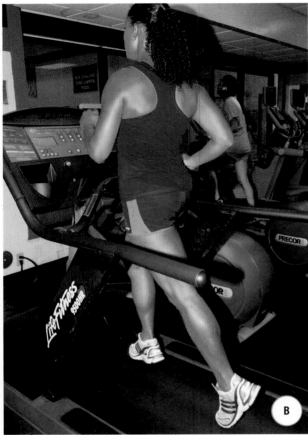

Treadmill running at a normal pace. Even on the treadmill, keep your gaze in front of you.

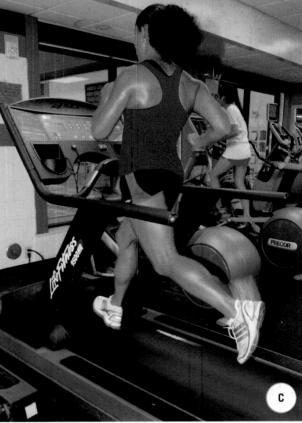

Running at an all-out sprint (T_2) pace. Notice the arms are higher and engaged.

ing a textbook style or that of some Olympic champion. The trouble with advocating a single best form is that everybody is different. Therefore, the safest, most effective improvement will come through evolving toward your own personal ideal that squeezes the most economy out of your body and your ergonomics.

How can you do this? It's easy: Run faster—and pay attention to what your body is doing as you run. In fact, says Carl, it's as simple as doing some sprints.

"Mother Nature is lazy and will find the easiest way to do things," he says. "That's why you can get away with stupid mechanics if you run slowly. But when you want to go faster, your mechanics will become more efficient."

If you want to see what "more efficient" looks like, have someone videotape you, ideally on a treadmill. First, run at a subthreshold (T_1) recovery pace **A**. Then, move up to your normal above-threshold (T_2) pace **B**. Then sprint **C**.

"You'll see better mechanics at above T_2 than sub T_1, and even better mechanics in the sprint," says Carl. "Sprinting is the best way to find your best form. It is not a surprise that sprinters have good mechanics to start with."

The bottom line is that you should listen to your own body.

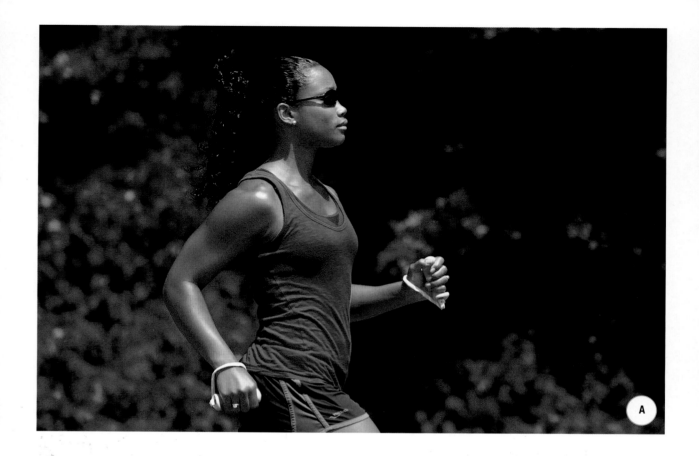

SALLY'S GOOD-FORM TIPS

In keeping with the philosophy that your form is your own business, Carl hesitates to say exactly what the elements of good form are. But I know what works for me. I've seen that you lose some sloppiness as you go faster. For me, good form includes the following:

- **Keep your head level and your neck straight.** Look 30 feet (9 m) ahead of you (which, incidentally, you can't do if you're running barefoot) to spot road obstacles.

- **Don't slump; run tall, with your shoulders aligned, spine straight, and chest open Ⓐ.** You get more oxygen into your body if your keep your shoulders back and expand your torso. Try it now while you are reading and notice how you breathe differently. Remember that you need to breathe freely, deeply, and rhythmically as you run.

- **Hands and arms should not cross the midline of your chest.** Hand position is not discussed much by anyone, but I think it's very important. The crossing of your chest, which is widespread among runners, is quite inefficient because it torques your body sideways. Sprinters generally don't do it, because they can't afford any left-to-right swaying that detracts from forward motion. You want a calm upper body. Hands should stay hip-width apart, in line with shoulders, swinging back and forth for light or energetic power on a vertical plane.

- **Get a Grip—actually, a pair of them.** A very useful tool I have found for reminding me to not cross my arms over my chest is a pair of e3 Grips, innovative, 2 oz (57 g) handgrips invented by a Sacramento, California, inventor friend of mine, Stephen Tamaribuchi. A Shiatsu massage therapist by trade who has become sort of a legend in these parts, Steve studied arm swing and found that a gripped hand position with a cocked thumb forces the arms into a vertical swing. I like the way the Grips make me focus on form rather than speed, distance, or breathing—just pure biomechanics. Chapter 11 has more information.

- **Keep your hands low when slow B, higher when fast C.** Arm and leg motions are linked, and match your arm action to your pace. Slower-paced long-distance runs require low energy expenditure, so keep your arms lower throughout their back-and-forth swinging motion. From the side view, your hands should look like they are moving back and forth, and up and down. While sprinting, when energy savings is not an issue, go ahead and vigorously push your arms/hands hard and high; this moves your legs faster.

- **Concentrate on the exhale.** I find that breathing out is very important for cleaning out the carbon dioxide, making room for fresh O_2, and improving lung capacity, respiratory rate, and inspired air volume. Avoiding a crossover arm swing will aid breathing.

- **Run light and try to work toward 180 strides per minute.** Eliminate heavy, shock-inducing, momentum-stopping footfalls. You are not a horse, clumping along at a heavy trot. Elite runners, known for their easy, fluid stride mechanics, are often counted in the neighborhood of 180 strides per minute. While I don't think I was ever that high and have certainly slowed as I've aged, I still do 167 strides per minute—a pace I like to match with the beats per minute. In fact, I developed an iTunes app called UpBeat Workouts to do that for me automatically.

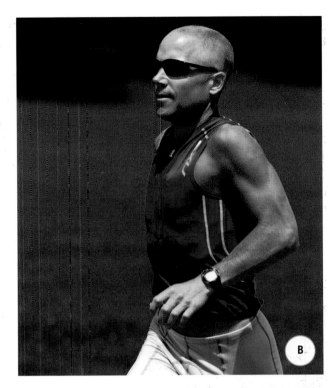

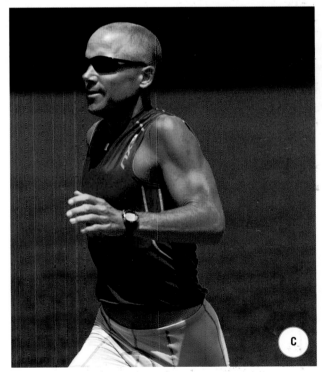

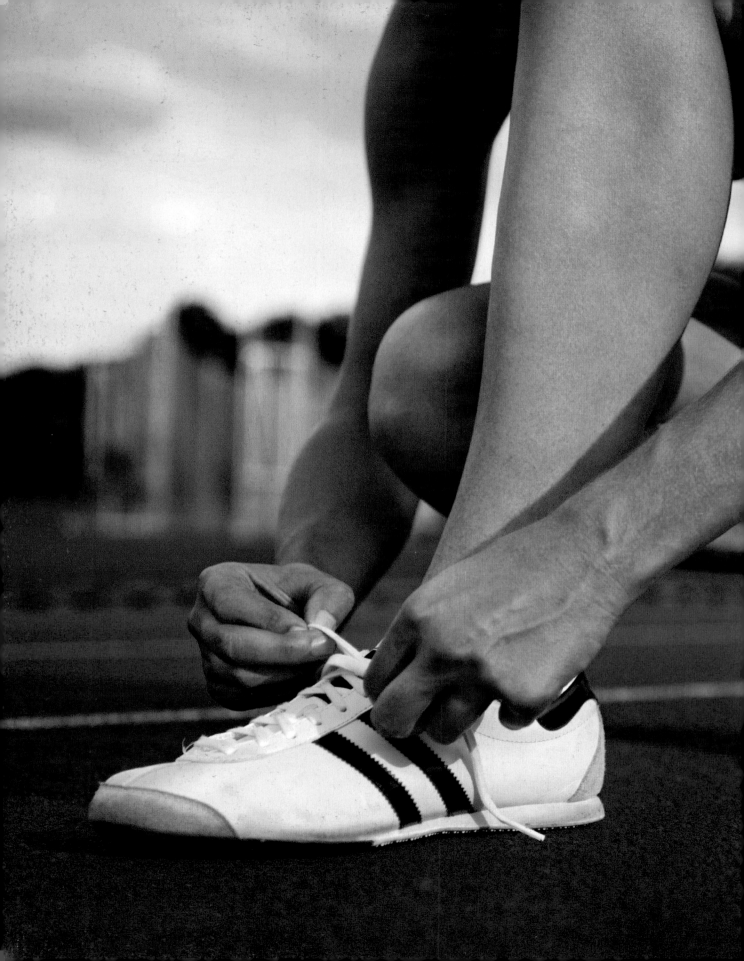

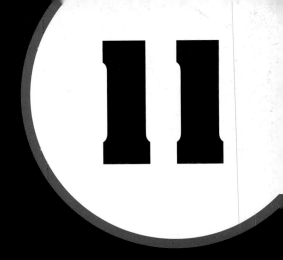

GET IN GEAR: THE LATEST APPAREL, SHOES, AND ACCESSORIES FOR EFFICIENT, COMFORTABLE RUNNING

I ADMIT IT—I'M A GEAR JUNKIE. When I go out and run nowadays, you might think I'm outfitted for combat. A Timex speed and distance monitor on one wrist, heart rate monitor on the other, dog leash holding my dog Adi Adi in one hand, water bottle strapped to the other, reflective vest on my torso, and fanny pack around my waist holding a cell phone, whistle, business card, money, energy bar, and dog biscuit. Inside my running shoes are orthotics. On my head, a baseball cap. When I run with training partners, I'll often have my hands clasped around e3 Grips, lightweight plastic hand forms that help give me a vertical arm swing (discussed later in this chapter).

You may think I'm obsessed and overdressed, but that's not true; every piece from head to toe is a functional necessity that makes my running more fun, safer, and more effective.

HOW FLEET FEET CAME TO LIFE

When I was in college, I had no idea I'd become a running-gear junkie, much less a running-business pioneer and a top-level athlete. My dream was to be a university athletics coach. But a fortuitous chain of circumstances landed me at the starting line of the running boom and the footwear technology explosion that came with it in the late 1970s. That gave me a first-hand view of new-product development and a clear understanding of the significance of having the right gear and the right fit every time you go out for a run. A little background:

Coaching had been my long-time career goal. And after getting my master's degree in kinesiology and physical education from Berkeley in 1970, serving as a Red Cross recreation volunteer in Vietnam for a year, and traveling before settling down to a intermediate school physical education teaching position and, finally, a coaching job at Monterey Peninsula College, it seems that I had achieved my dream. The trouble was that it only lasted a year. At that college and many others in the era before Title 9, female coaches were hired only for short stints to preserve jobs for male coaches. So, at age twenty-six, I was back on the street, trying to figure out what to do with the rest of my life.

Then I ran into Elizabeth Jansen, who was my best friend through high school. We met in eighth grade and started playing tennis together after I bought some feed for a cow I was raising from her father, the owner of Walter Jansen & Sons Feed and Grain. Hanging around, Elizabeth picked up some business tips by osmosis. Now newly divorced, she was still playing some serious tennis. Since I was falling in love with running—actually winning a lot of races, including the longest one in the area, the Lakes at the Pines 10-miler (16.1 km)—I came up with a business proposal: Since we both needed to make a living and both had a hard time finding good athletic shoes at Goodwin and Cole, the local sporting goods store in Sacramento, California, why not start an athletic shoe store?

Elizabeth came up with the name Fleet Feet.

Now, keep in mind that this was a fairly radical idea at the time. Back then, there was no athletic shoe store in Sacramento or the entire region. In fact, no one even knew what an athletic shoe store was.

In 1976, there was no Foot Locker in the mall. There was no Athlete's Foot. There was only our stand-alone Fleet Feet Sports in a tumbledown, Victorian two-story next to a vacant lot in a run-down part of mid-town. We paid $22,000 for the abandoned house, which only survived the bulldozers because it was declared a historical landmark. We slept in the living room and a bedroom, using the dining room and the parlor room with the big picture window facing J Street as the store.

Getting the right gear wasn't an issue for us at Fleet Feet; getting any gear was. For inventory, we borrowed $20,000 from the only bank that would lend us money (thanks, River City Bank!), but Puma and Adidas, the two big brands at the time, wouldn't sell to us. Eventually, we stocked the shelves with product from Converse and Osaga, an Oregon-based brand which used a Japanese name for marketing cache, and started selling wrestling shoes, football cleats, tennis shoes, and running shoes. Back then, the latter did not have female models.

Fleet Feet was by no means an instant success. To get the word out, we bought a big postal van, painted it bright yellow, and showed up with shoes and tables at races thrown by the Buffalo Chips Running Club, Sacramento's first running club (and yes, named after buffalo dung). Business was slow; it was a big deal in 1976 if 100 people showed up to a race. It took months to get sales up to $100 a day—that was five pairs of shoes.

It took a year to get sales up to $200 a day. That's not a lot, but it was an important benchmark because it let us pick up Adidas and Puma—and business surged. Soon we were up to $500 a day and decided to open a second store in Chico, a college town of 75,000 about 100 miles north (161 km) of Sacramento.

THE RISE OF MODERN RUNNING GEAR

The shoes in the mid-1970s were nothing like we have now. The Osagas came in three different models and colors, all with nylon uppers and a thin sole with no EVA padding. The Adidas and Pumas weren't much different. That abruptly started to change in 1978 when we picked up Nike, which had been growing rapidly since it introduced the Waffle Trainer in 1974.

Created when Nike co-founder and University of Oregon track coach Bill Bowerman poured liquid urethane into his wife's waffle iron in search of a grippier outsole, the Waffle Trainer was a sensation. People loved the cushioning it provided. We had waiting lists for them. The other brands rushed to come up with their own cushioning.

Thankfully, the shoe companies finally began making a small assortment of women's running shoes built on women's lasts (discussed shortly) and in women's colors. Nike's Lady Cortez, the first women's shoe we carried, was a huge hit. It was narrower and built on research based on the morphology of a woman's foot, so it naturally fit better. We no longer had to take a men's size and subtract by 1.5 so that women could wear men's shoes.

Then, like clockwork, dual-density foam arrived. Then shoes for pronators and supinators (defined shortly) arrived. Nike introduced the Tailwind, with its flared heel and less-knobby waffle soles, and then debuted the technology that changed everything: Air. Nike Air—a cushioning pocket in the heel, filled with a secret. That unleashed a wave of competing technologies. The cushioning revolution was on.

I believe these innovations and the others that have followed truly have helped runners perform better and get injured less often. They also allowed runners to customize shoes just for themselves, for their own feet and own biomechanics. Personally, I loved it. With my bunions, bowed legs, and attention to biomechanics, this was a dream.

Before the late 1970s, shoe stores had been concerned only with fit, using polished chrome Branock devices to measure length and width. Then, as the new technologies came on-line, we had to learn about function and concepts such as "support" and "control."

Competition grew fierce. When the national chains such as Foot Locker moved into the local malls, and other running shoe stores began popping up, Fleet Feet fought back by specializing in customer service, building in-store club houses where runners could hang out, sponsoring races, holding seminars, opening more stores and franchising our brand, and, of course, carrying the gear and accessories that people were asking for.

Being a competitive runner, I was also a roving market researcher. After my knee collapsed at mile 20 (km 32) of my first marathon, the Silver State marathon in Reno, Nevada, in 1977 (I walked the last 6 miles [9.7 km] and finished in 4:07), I got orthotics. By 1980, moving up from 50-milers (80 km) to the Western States 100, I was well versed in reflective clothing, straps, vests, hydration devices, sunglasses, lace locks, insoles, and lots of apparel—hats, gloves, and rain gear (but not heart rate monitors, which were still five years away). At Fleet Feet, we even carried something called Shoe Goo, sole-repair putty that would fill in holes and worn sections to extend the life of the $20 shoe.

Since I sold the forty-store Fleet Feet Sports franchise and several of my own retail locations in 1993, the quantity and sophistication of running shoes and accessories has continued to grow. And that's part of the intrigue of the sport—figuring out what pair of shorts or speed and distance monitor works for you. Following is a comprehensive list of the products I have found to be essential for any runner, starting with a primer on the most technical and universal of all running products, shoes.

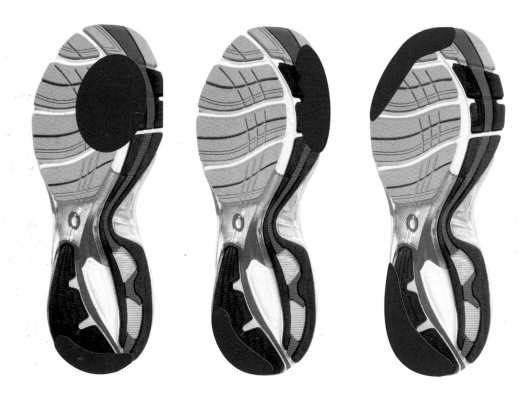

Wear test: The patches represent wear on the bottom worn by shoe of a neutral pronator.

THE RUNNING SHOE PRIMER

Are you a pronator or a supinator? Do you need a neutral shoe, a motion-control shoe, a cushioned-stability shoe, a combination-lasted shoe?

Confused? Don't be embarrassed if you are. Running certainly is loaded with its own lingo, and nothing about the sport may be more complicated than the types, parts, and construction of shoes, the foundation of your running ensemble. Despite the colorful debate nowadays over whether you need to run in cushioned shoes, uncushioned shoes, or no shoes at all (see the discussion of barefoot

running in Chapter 10), my crystal ball tells me that most runners like and benefit from the cushioning, stabilization, and protection of running shoes and will continue to wear them for the foreseeable future. So, if you want to know what varieties are out there (cushioned, cushioned-stability, stability), who they are made for (overpronators, supinators, neutral runners), what's right for you, and what the heck those magazine reviews are talking about, read on. No one shoe fits everybody the same, but after this, you'll understand what category is most appropriate for your foot's unique biomechanics.

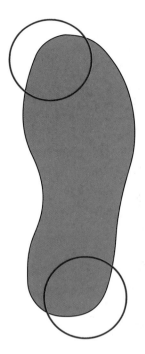
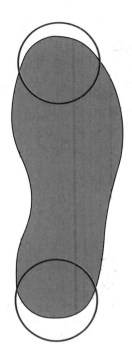
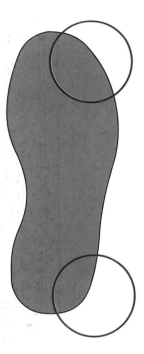

Wear test: The bottom circles represent wear on the shoe of an over pronator.

REMEMBER THAT PRONATION IS GOOD

Before anything else, realize that pronation is not a bad thing. It's actually normal, the body's response to the impact forces incurred when your foot hits the ground during running and walking. At impact, the arch elongates and flattens and the foot rolls inward to help absorb shock.

Problems occur when there is too much or not enough pronation—resulting in less shock absorption by the foot itself and bone misalignment that can, over time, transfer more of this impact stress to the joints, tendons, and muscles. The culprit may be a too-flexible arch or a too-stiff arch, the former belonging to an overpronator and the latter to a supinator (underpronator).

TAKE TWO TESTS: WEAR TEST AND BATHROOM TEST

Before you get to know the shoes, you must get to know your feet. Two simple tests will help you do this: the wear test, which requires a quick glance at your shoes, and the bathroom test, which requires a quick look at your footprints when you get out of the shower.

• **Wear test:** Take your running shoes and turn them over. The bottoms, the wear markings on your outer sole, tell you as much about your running style as a video camera that tries to capture your biomechanical patterns. If your shoe shows acute wear on the outside of the heel, general wear in the forefoot emanating out from the ball of the foot, and little to no wear on the outside and

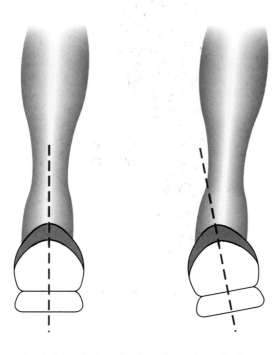

Wear test: The bottom of a shoe of a supinator (underpronator)

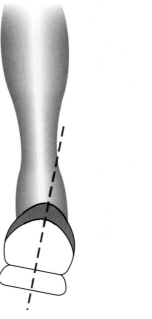
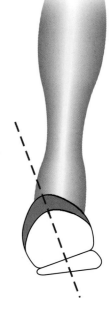

Wear test: Heel strikes for neutral, overpronation, supination, and severe overpronation

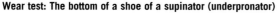

inside edges of the shoe, you have a neutral wear pattern and normal pronation. If the wear pattern is greater on the inside of the shoe, you're an overpronator; if it's greater on the outside of the shoe, you're a supinator.

- **Bathroom test:** Get your feet wet and stand normally. You're normal/neutral if your footprints do not include most of the medial zone, where the arch is located. However, if your footprint is solid from heel to toe, with no cutaway where a normal arch would be, it

means your foot flattens out too much and you're an overpronator. If your footprint overemphasizes the outer edge of your foot and leaves a huge open space from the arch area, indicting that you may have a rigid arch that doesn't flatten much, you're a supinator.

Ideally, when your foot flattens and rolls too much or not enough, the proper shoe or insole can straighten things out.

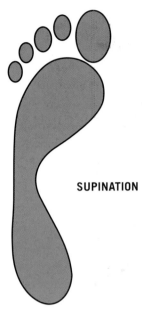

SUPINATION

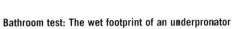

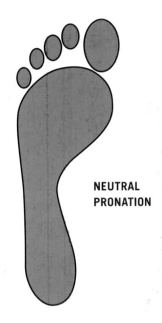

NEUTRAL PRONATION

Bathroom test: The wet footprint of an underpronator

Bathroom test: The wet footprint of a neutral pronator

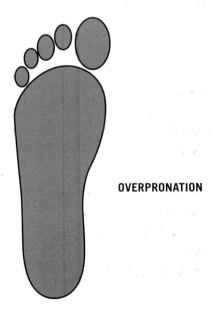

OVERPRONATION

Bathroom test: The wet footprint of an overpronator

MATCH YOUR FEET TO YOUR CORRECT SHOES

Here's how to match your feet to your correct shoes.

Pronator (Neutral Foot Striker)

Humans are supposed to pronate. Pronation is a normal gait cycle: a landing on the outer portion of the heel; and inward roll that disperses shock by flattening the foot and puts the entire forefoot in contact with the ground (allowing complete, balanced support of your body weight); and finally, a very slight outward roll that results in a fairly even push-off from the front of the foot, with the big toe pushing off last. It is thought that 30 percent to 40 percent of runners have this normal pronation.

Preferred shoes and biomechanical suggestions: Wear a neutral cushioned shoe or a cushion-stability trainer, which will not detract from your natural gait. Avoid motion-control shoes with serious stability/controlling devices, such as a medial post.

Overpronator

The foot of an overpronator makes initial ground contact with the outside of the heel, and then rolls inward too much, moving too far to the medial side. Look for excessive wear on the inner side of your running shoes and a tilt inward when placed on a flat surface.

Overpronation is a potential problem because the foot is still rolling when it should be pushing off, so it pushes off unevenly, making the big toe and second toe do all the work. This twists and strains the foot, ankle, and knee as they struggle to stabilize the body and absorb shock. It also can cause tightness in muscles that are forced to compensate to align and stabilize those joints. Overpronation is associated with overly flexible arches and muscle strength imbalances. It is generally thought that most runners have some degree of overpronation.

Preferred shoes and biomechanical suggestions: Wear a firm, inflexible shoe in the motion-control or stability category. These will limit the inward roll of the foot with external and internal support devices, such as a medial post (a plastic post and/or firm, denser foam under the medial side of the arch) and a straighter-than-usual last (the shape of the shoe). Orthotics devices or arch supports can be used as well; add a cushioned insole if you want a softer ride. Spend some extra time stretching, too.

Supinator

Also referred to as underpronation, supination is the opposite of pronation—the lack of an inward roll across the forefoot after the initial landing on the outer portion of the heel. Look for excessive wear along the entire outside edge of your running shoes, from heel to toe—not just at the heel. A supinator's shoes will tilt outward when placed on a flat surface.

A rare condition (no more than 5 percent of runners have it), supination occurs when the foot remains on its lateral (outside) edge from impact to push-off, concentrating force and weight in a relatively small sector of the foot and forcing the smaller toes to do most of the push-off work at the end of the cycle. This lack of normal pronation increases injury risk because it minimizes the foot's ability to dissipate shock well, and puts impact forces on smaller bones of the foot that lack the tensile strength to handle foot strike. (That's one of the reasons the big toe and the first metatarsal are the thickest and strongest of the toes and small foot bones, respectively.)

Preferred shoes and biomechanical suggestions: Do not wear a stability shoe. Wear a lightweight shoe in the cushioned or neutral category that has significant flexibility on the medial side (inner edge) and a curved last; that will encourage pronation (inward foot motion). Since a tight Achilles tendon and other leg muscles and connective tissues contribute to supination, do extra stretching for the calves, hamstrings, quads, and iliotibial band.

REVIEWING THE TYPES OF SHOES

Motion-Control Shoes

Designed to protect against overpronation, these heavy, expensive, inflexible shoes are loaded with control and stability features, including a medial post and a straight last. They are all about support and durability.

Stability or Structured Trainers

These shoes, used by the majority of runners, are halfway between motion-control and neutral shoes. They often have a dual-density midsole (two different materials for different compressions) to reduce overpronation.

Lightweight Cushioned or Neutral Trainers

Traditionally known as cushioned, but often now supplanted by the term "neutral," these shoes lack any medial or rearfoot stability devices, and are preferred by runners who have good form and by supinators.

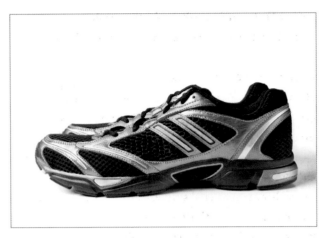

Motion control running shoes

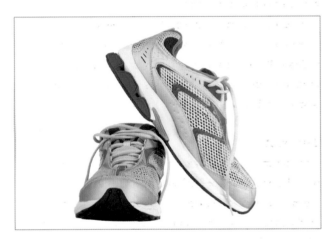

Stability or structured trainers

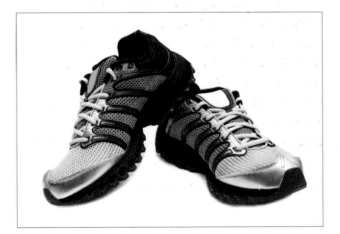

Lightweight cushion traniers

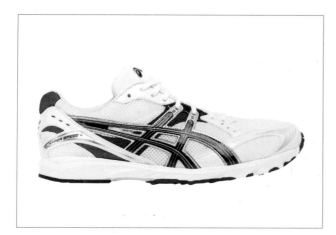

Racing flats

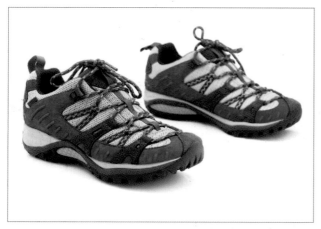

Train runners

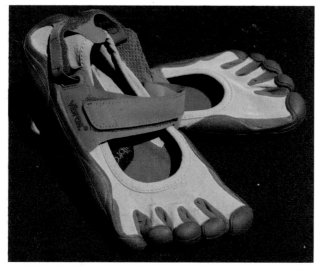

Primal-Gait shoes

Racing Flats

Ultra-light and über-flexible race-day shoes, these minimalist, barely cushioned dogs, often worn without socks, are designed for lightweight, elite runners who run fast—near or under forty-minute 10Ks and three-hour marathons. They are close to primal-gait/barefoot running shoes (see the "Primal-Gait Shoes" section) because there is no cushion, there is little support, and they allow the foot to travel after foot strike however it chooses to move. They are faster on race day because you have lower energy cost with the lower weight that you carry on your foot.

Trail Runners

With a hard rubber sole from front to back (not in spots like regular trainers), deep treads, and a tough, often water-resistant exterior, trail runners have the extra durability, traction, and stability needed on rough, uneven dirt trails. Some are cut higher around the ankle to seal out trail debris; optional, add-on gaitors will do the same thing. Regular shoes can work well on trails, but these will hold up longer in repeated off-road use.

Primal-Gait Shoes

This emerging category of minimalist running footwear with little or no cushioning or structure debuted in 2004 with the Nike Free, and has come to include barefoot shoes such as the Vibram Five Fingers. All of them attempt to discourage a heel-strike landing and encourage a forefoot landing, which you would naturally do when running bare-foot. The primal-gait category also includes new, highly engineered shoes such as Newton, which use specially designed uneven footbeds that attempt to force you into a forefoot landing.

The Parts of the Shoe

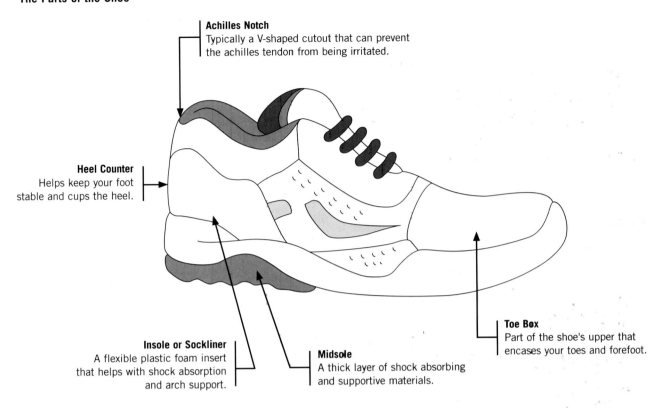

Achilles Notch
Typically a V-shaped cutout that can prevent the achilles tendon from being irritated.

Heel Counter
Helps keep your foot stable and cups the heel.

Insole or Sockliner
A flexible plastic foam insert that helps with shock absorption and arch support.

Midsole
A thick layer of shock absorbing and supportive materials.

Toe Box
Part of the shoe's upper that encases your toes and forefoot.

CONSTRUCTION ZONE: THE PARTS OF THE SHOE

To figure out what shoe is best for your foot, it'll help to know what you're getting into. A running shoe is a remarkably complex housing for athletic feet on the move, designed to protect and propel you, too often diametrically opposed functions. Here's how the component pieces work together to get the job done.

The Last, but Not Least

Derived from the Old English word "laest," or footprint, the last is the basic shape of a shoe: straight, curved, or semicurved. The last technically is the three-dimensional mold that the shoe is built around, like a pattern. Semi-curved is easily the best seller, used by runners with normal pronation. As mentioned earlier, to control inward roll, overpronators use an inflexible shoe with a straight last, which does not indent much at the arch. Conversely, a curved last encourages supinators to roll inward; also, most racing shoes are built on a curved last.

- **Elastic shoelaces or lace locks:** Securing your running shoes snugly can prevent injuries as well as blisters. My running partner, Cathy Anderson-Myers, tripped and fell hard on concrete when her shoelaces accidentally came untied. Better to choose a pair of lace locks or elastic shoelaces.

SAFETY, FORM, AND HYDRATION ACCESSORIES

Regardless of your fitness and the miles you've run, you can literally be tripped up by poor housekeeping and planning. Just as you wouldn't expect to drive 300 miles (483 km) on a quarter of a tank of gas, you could crash and burn by ignoring safety.

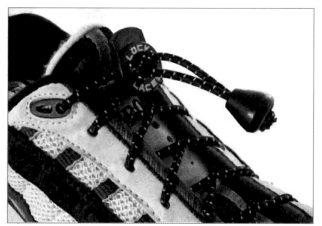

Lace Locks

- **Lace locks:** There's no reason to have an untied lace trip you up. Cheap and effective, they cinch your laces tightly and lock them instantly in place. Elastic laces may be your preference, although I find they can create pressure on top of your foot.
- **e3 Grips:** These ingenious 2 oz (57 g) hand forms—invented by my long-time friend, Sacramento, California, coach and Shiatsu massage therapist Stephen Tamaribuchi—help give you a classic vertical arm swing. They work by positioning your fingers in a way that pulls your elbow into your side, eliminating the inefficient chest crossover of a normal arm swing. I noticed an improvement in my form immediately and have used them for years, as have many of my running chums. I love them for one more reason: They keep my focus on my biomechanics. Even after forty years of running, I want to be a more efficient runner and this is one of the best ways that I know to accomplish that.
- **Road ID:** Attached to a runner's shoe, this waterproof, reflective, emergency/medical ID tag instantly provides your name, brief medical history, and emergency contact information to anyone who picks your injured body up off the street. If you prefer, check out the bracelet version of this ID which comes with an identification number that provides emergency responders with all of the information about your medical history.

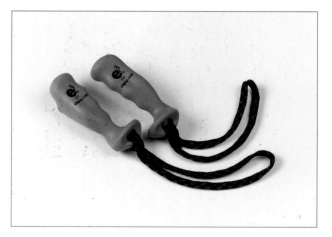

e3 Grips

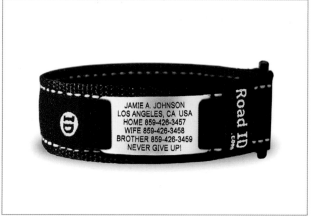

Road ID

- **Hydration fanny pack:** These hip-hugging, zippered cargo belts from Amphipod, Camelbak, Ultimate Direction, and other good brands carry one, two, or more bottles of fluid, making them essential for long runs, trail runs, and anyone who needs his or her own special mix. They're great for carrying MP3 players and food, too. Tip: Make sure the bottles hold tight in their holsters and don't bounce as you run. Hand-held bottles with built-in hold-straps also work well, but can throw off the pace of faster runners unless you change hands often.

- **Roller-massager:** Nothing rubs away your post-run muscle strains and stiffness like these popular twenty-first-century rollers from companies such as The Stick and MuscleTrac. They're great for pre-race warm-ups, too. Pamper yourself—five minutes of this self-massage per day will be a relief and a pure pleasure.

- **Nip guards:** Hey, it's a guy thing. These tiny, sweat-proof, adhesive bandage disks protect men's nipples from abrasion and bleeding caused by rubbing against a shirt during long runs. If you have ever seen a man running along with two vertical stripes of blood staining the front of his singlet, you know he's in agony and swearing that he'll use nipple protection next time.

- **Lube:** Last but not least is this often-forgotten chafe fighter, which can made a difference between a fun day at the races and an agonizing death march. Many brands are available. Before the race begins, put it where the sun don't shine—underarms and under there—and you'll cross the finish line smiling.

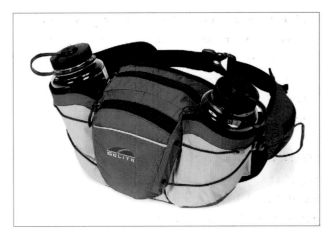

Hydration fanny pack

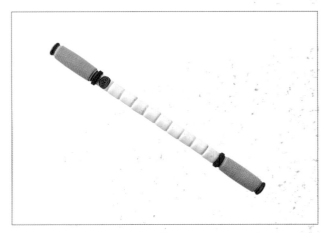

The Stick massager

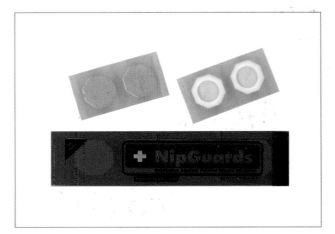

Nip Guards

WINDOW INTO THE FUTURE: APPLICATION SOFTWARE

Using software to make you a better runner isn't new; the original runner's software first hit the scenes with Jim and Laurie Dotter's PC Coach in the early 1990s and was quickly followed by logging software from Athlete's Diary. But today's new breed of software has upped the ante. The latest from the Canadian company Dynastream is a way to have all of your tools become interoperable—that is, talk to each other. The transmission protocol called ANT+ (pronounced "ant plus") allows your heart rate monitor from Timex to talk to your receiver from Garmin that can connect to your Suunto foot pod or your Saris Power Tap on your bike. And all of that data from the different tools—the power meter, heart rate monitor, and bike computer—can send the data to your mobile phone which sends it to a website of your choice that stores it for you. Check out the Adidas MiCoach app, Wahoo fitness app, Nike Training, Runkeeper, or Runmeter for your mobile device. And, if you are into the next step, share. Share this information with your running friends using any social web site that tells your friends where you are, what route you just ran, what music you liked, what your run was like, and who you ran with.

And, I love these technologies that automatically, without any effort from you, do it seamlessly. For me, it's like the icing on the cake; I love it. For example, how important is it for you to know during or after your run that you were running 9 mph (14.5 kph); you have 3.7 miles (6 km) to go; you hit the power music button five times to energize yourself; your total ascent was 500 yards (457 m); your accurate burn rate based on your metabolic tests was 75 percent carbohydrate, 20 percent fat, and 5 percent protein compared to your last run, when your carb burn rate was 65 percent; your sweat rate and hydration levels maintained themselves; your elapsed time was 75 minutes; you ran your favorite course thirty seconds faster than you did a week ago; it was an upbeat workout; your average strides per minute were 165 and average heart rate was 162 . . . should I continue?

As for the platform, I recommend ENKIsports.com app and web platform, which costs about $5 per month for the tools and look for the ANT+ logo on your devices which means that they can all connect to each other and allows you the ability to relay your data and position to one central point that stores the info in a way that you or your coach can access it and make suggestions. You can know if you are above the training intensity in prescribed watts or heart beats. With the GPS-enabled device, you have mapping functions (so that if you get lost you can get back easily). You can see if you are doing better this run from last month's run.

What's in the future is even more exciting than what we have today. We'll have devices that not only measure and monitor our running, but also manage it in a way that we can compare, contrast, and see trends: Are we getting stronger, faster, and more efficient? New smart fabrics will someday eliminate the discomfort of a transmitter belt and wireless devices in our shoes will tell us our foot-strike impact and function, which will do away with the need for the bathroom test, see page 162.

Computer chips in shoes failed the first time, but they will certainly return someday, giving both elite and everyday runners information on their type of insole as well as the wear and tear on the outer and mid sole materials. And it'll be safer, too. These technologies and platforms will reduce the number of injuries, increase the enjoyment, and provide ways for us to run together with each other or virtually without effort, and all of this will be bundled into fewer and fewer devices. Someday, you will not have to spend five minutes before your run setting up your Garmin to find a satellite (speed, distance, location monitor), setting your Timex or Bion Blink (the flashing zone heart rate monitor) to set your zones for the workout, your Blackberry or iPhone to find the right app, your MP3 player that auto connects your strides per minute with your music or your bpm of your heart rate or song. What a wonderful running world it will be when the training tool, the device, does all of this for you, automatically, with only the tap of your finger and only take a nanosecond of time to synchronize.

Did you think that running was a simple matter of lacing up a pair of shoes and throwing on some old clothes that you had lying around in your chest of drawers? Did you think that running is boring or that only boring people run? There is running the old way and there is running the new way. It's time to test-drive the modern-day running gear that makes it possible to run farther, faster, and in less time.

Nothing I just discussed in this chapter is a gadget or a throwaway item. This is essential gear to provide you with the Three Es of running: enjoyment, energy, and efficiency (well, maybe it needs to be four Es, as entertainment needs to be in there somewhere).

How does it look and feel to have the right shoes to match your gait, the right safety gear to meet your conditions, the right training tools to improve and enhance your performance? It looks good and feels great. It's an entirely new way to run with the same old training partners, whether they are four-legged or two-legged.

Treat yourself. Go to your local running store, try something new, and go through the different phases with a smile as you struggle with getting it to work, learning how to use it, and adjusting to the changes. Whether it is custom orthotics or a massage stick, the right gear will make a difference and keep you on the roads, on the trails, or running—even if it's in the swimming pool when you turn 100 years old.

>>> Tips for Mobile Device Tools

The new running tools loaded on your mobile device are time-saving and provide you with robust feedback information on your workout. Here are some quick tips if you love and use them like I do.

1. GPS only works outdoors; accelerometer foot pods work anywhere.
2. Get an armband to carry your mobile device. Throwing it in your pocket or snapping it on a waistband simply don't work as well.
3. Set up a running playlist of music that matches your tempo. When you match your running cadence with your music tempo, you'll discover the time goes by faster and, well, the research shows you run faster too. Check out "Upbeat Workouts" (page 171) as a resource.

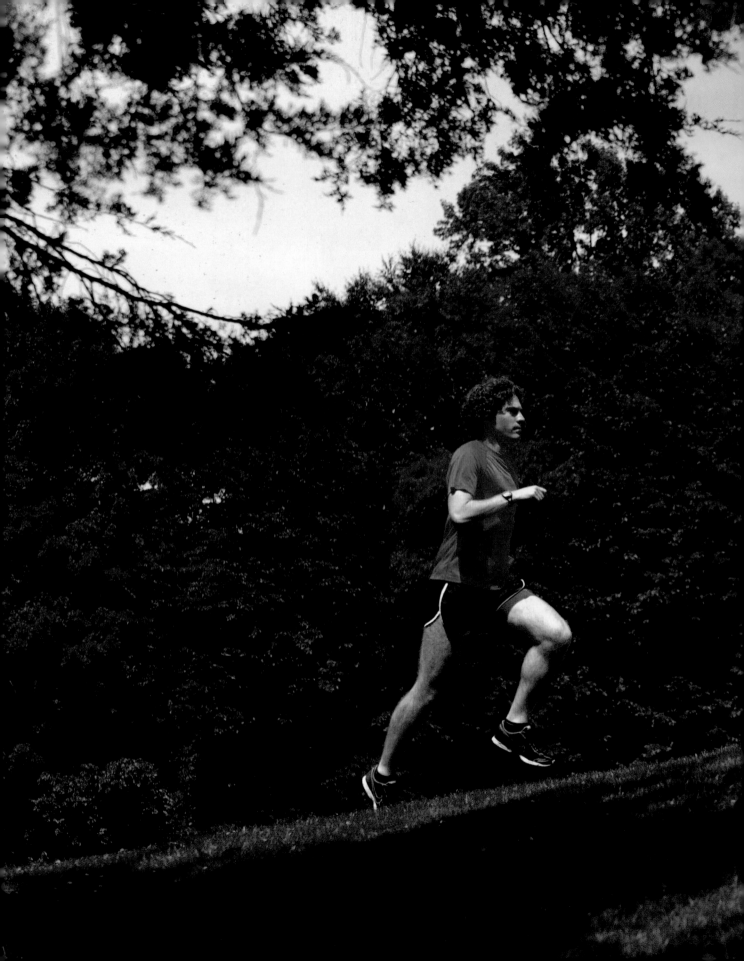

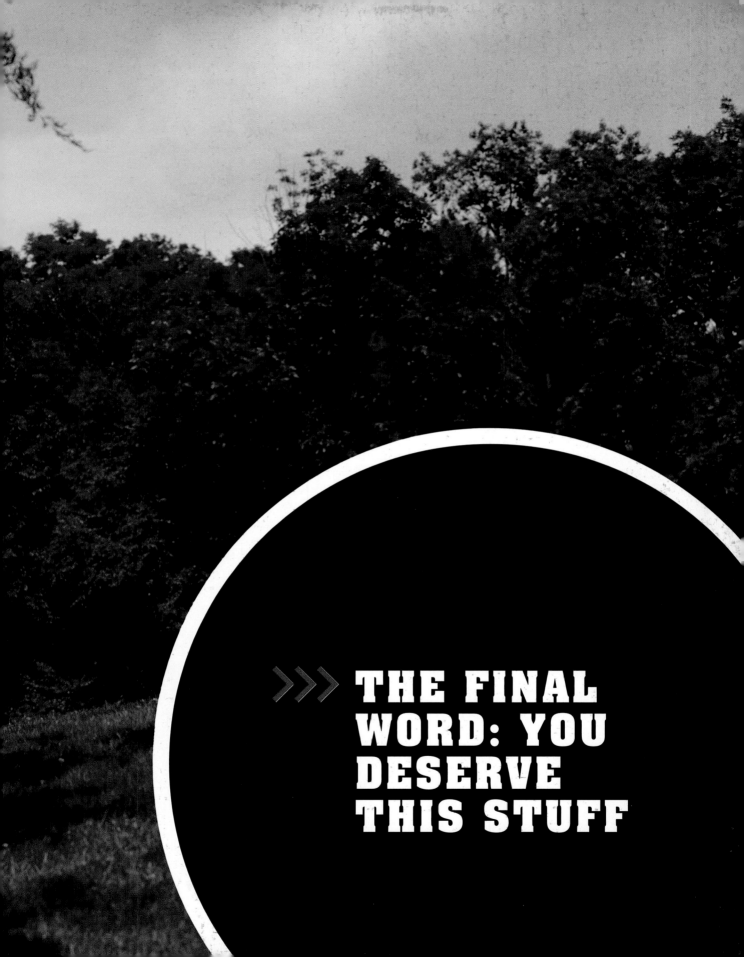

>>> THE FINAL WORD: YOU DESERVE THIS STUFF

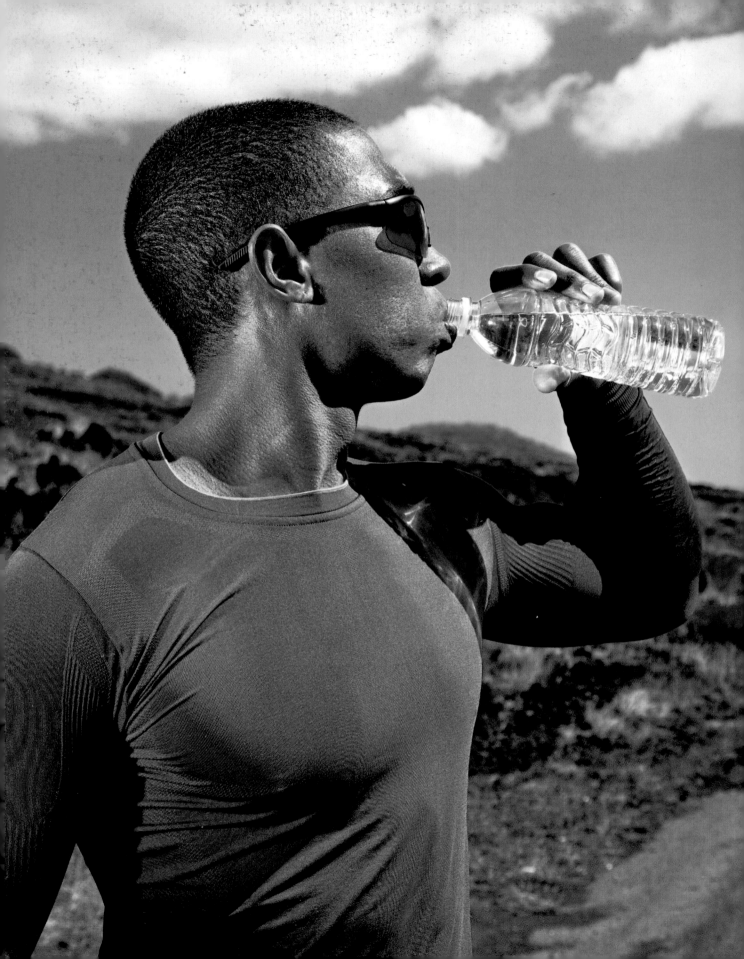

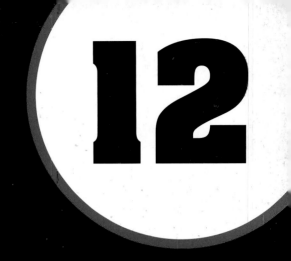

NUTRITION AND HYDRATION: EAT AND DRINK FOR OPTIMAL HEALTH AND PERFORMANCE

YOU MIGHT THINK the question most often asked during my lectures and via email would be, "Sally, how can I run better and faster?"—or perhaps, "How do I fall in love with running like you have?" After all, my body of work focuses almost entirely on answering such questions. However, I am continually surprised by the actual question that I am asked most often: "What should I eat?" It seems that the need for nutritional information and dietary suggestions is enormous.

Fortunately, the answer to the simple question—what should I eat?—can also be rather simple, although many new runners imagine that there must be some secret, special kind of food. There isn't, and the simple answer is: eat healthy, real food. How simple this really is depends in part on your current diet and knowledge of nutrition. But keep in mind that the more you run the more you can eat—with one important caveat: as long as you fuel well. The suggestions and guidelines provided in this chapter should make fueling well for your runs and your best health much easier, even if you are already eating healthy now.

Over the years as a competitive endurance athlete, I have determined the best food, drinks, and supplements to fuel my muscles and maintain my high energy level. Along the way, I've tested scores of nutritional plans and dietary suggestions, forming my own conclusions about what works. My bookshelves once overflowed with books on diet and nutrition. I say "once" because, after researching and writing about diet and exercise for decades, I finally let go of several dozen texts to make room for new ones. Conventional wisdom about food has been changing fast.

Way back in 1976, when my partner Elizabeth Jansen and I started Fleet Feet Sports, we sold books for runners on what, how often, and why to eat. They were heavily weighted toward an old myth about calories—calories in equals calories out—that I'll disprove in this chapter. Knowledge has improved as the times have changed; in the mid-1970s, the United States didn't face an obesity epidemic or such a widespread incidence of diseases from lethargy. Not yet on the map was knowledge about such things as the importance of nonexercise activity thermogenesis, or "NEAT," (see the "NEAT-ness Counts!" sidebar), a new calculation for and understanding of calorie-burning nonexercise movements, and the relationship of eating and emotions was rarely discussed and even less understood.

In the 1970s, a notion popularized by many of the runners of that time, including Boston Marathon legend Bill Rogers, was that if you run, you can eat anything. Back then, there were no scientifically engineered foods or drink formulas that optimize gastric dumping. The words "energy drink" weren't even in our vocabulary. I'll never forget the time my running buddies and I holed up in the kitchen with ground-up bee pollen, table salt, aspirin, and Coke, trying to concoct a magic formula to solve the equation of ingesting simple calories in liquid form. Too often, during a long, hot 75- or 100-mile (121 or 161 km) run, my stomach would revolt, shutting down the pyloric sphincter and preventing fluids from passing into my intestines. The result was nasty: an awful stomach bloating and pain, nausea, and throwing up.

>>> NEAT-ness Counts!

Researchers from the Mayo Clinic have discovered a new trick to fire up your metabolism: nonexercise activity thermogenesis, or "NEAT." NEAT includes all the little movements that make up our day. Not the big movements such as exercise, and not the motionlessness of sitting still or deep sleep. NEAT activities include standing (rather than sitting), fidgeting, walking around, shopping, cleaning, gardening, and playing the guitar.

Why does NEAT matter? Well, according to research findings published in *Science Magazine* obese persons sit, on average, 150 minutes more each day than their leaner counterparts. This means obese people burn 350 fewer NEAT calories per day than do lean people.

To detect even the smallest tap of the toe, Mayo Clinic researchers invented a monitoring system incorporating technology used in fighter-jet control panels. They embedded sensors in customized, data-logging undergarments. Their conclusion: Obese people are NEAT-deficient. While it's unclear why, in the meantime, keep those fingers tapping and those toes wiggling. To read more, go to www.sciencemag.org.

What I would do if starting over, and what I urge anyone truly serious about mapping out a new health and fitness plan for themselves, is to get professional nutritional advice from a registered dietician (RD)—some even specialize in sports nutrition. A professional consultation with an RD or similar professional could streamline your transition to lifelong success and healthy living.

FIND HEALTHY FOODS YOU LIKE

These days, few athletes can be found in their kitchens, whipping up experimental energy potions. The choice of pre-packaged energy bars, drinks, and supplements is endless and growing. Unfortunately, many of them are heavily laced with artificial flavoring, artificial stimulants, and artificial results. I think we can do better.

While there is no single list or criterion for the best foods to fuel your running activities—you still must experiment to find the right combination of foods for your body, needs, and tastes—reducing the clutter to analyze the foods available to determine what will work best for you is possible.

The first rule—whether you are a runner, a weight lifter, or an auto mechanic—is eat healthy. Whole, natural, nutrient-rich foods not only promote good general health and reduce disease risks, but also provide complete and wholesome sources of energy. These foods include fruits and vegetables families, rich omega 3 and 6 seafood, eggs and dairy, beans and legumes, and lean poultry and meat. If you are a vegetarian like I am you can easily replace meats with nuts and seeds. Healthy foods rounding out the list include minimally processed grains, spices and herbs, natural sweeteners such as honey and molasses, and drinks such as green tea and fresh-filtered water.

What combination of the aforementioned foods is right for you? I can only tell you what I found to be right for me and how I arrived at it. Four decades ago, venturing into some of the toughest running, biking, and swimming events in the endurance world, I began experimenting with diet and nutrition, noting what worked for me. I challenge you to do the same. Set your criteria, develop your list of foods, and measure and test your responses. At the end of the day, the week, the race, ask the key question about energy and performance: Did I do better?

The key criteria I use can be summarized as follows:

- **The healthiest foods for me provide more energy.** I want to feel light after eating, fueled but not full, more awake and not weighted down. I eat for energy—both emotional and physical energy.

- **The healthiest foods for me are the most nutrient-dense.** I choose foods rich in the essential nutrients—the most vitamins, minerals, phytonutrients, essential fatty acids, fiber, etc. for the least number of calories. Nutrient-dense foods promote optimal health because their nutrient level is so high in relation to the number of calories they contain.

- **The healthiest foods for me are whole foods.** These foods are not highly processed, and contain no synthetic, irradiated, or artificial ingredients. I prefer organically grown foods since they contain no pesticides and have a reduced impact on the earth—it's as much about being good for the planet as it is about good food for me.

- **The healthiest foods for me are ones that are easy to get.** I have a list of familiar, everyday foods that I can gather efficiently from local markets—fruits, vegetables, and breads that don't require a lot of time for shopping, cooking, or preparing.

- **The healthiest foods for me are the best quality and freshest.** I like to eat seasonal foods that are locally grown and affordable.

- **The healthiest foods for me are the ones that match my tastes.** I like to eat foods that taste good to me. Surprising to many friends, chocolate is not one of those.

Once your criteria are set and you've figured out what foods to include and exclude from your menu, the next step is determining what, when, and how much to eat. Again, I recommend consulting to help perfect your nutritional and dietary plan. To provide simplified criteria for healthy food selection, I used the same structure that has worked so well in training: zones. But instead of aerobic/anaerobic heart rate training zones, I set up a guide to dietary zones.

THINK IN TERMS OF FOOD ZONES: SEPARATING HEALTHY FOODS FROM UNHEALTHY FOODS

Walking into any grocery store, we are confronted with a vast landscape of dietary choices, seemingly growing by the hour. Even after figuring out what to eat, honing it down to metabolically sound, high-energy products that are practical and affordable, there are numerous decisions to make about quantity, quality, selection, packaging, availability, preparation, and when, where, and how often to eat.

BECOMING ACQUAINTED WITH THE FOOD ZONES CHART

My approach to all aspects of life—business, athletic, emotional, etc.—is always to simplify, and food is no different. To simplify food choices, I developed a chart—the Food Zones Chart **(see Figure 12.1)**. It helps make the seemingly complex issue of "What should I eat?" as simple as looking at a index card.

The chart employs the zones concept that should be familiar to you by now. It includes five different Food Zones and a threshold, represented by the white line between Zones 4 and 5. Instead of zones by heart rate, these zones are, of course, defined by foods. The zones range from healthiest (Zone 1) to toxic (Zone 5), and the foods in the zones are evaluated and numbered by their metabolic load—the impact of that food on your vital physiological processes.

Zone 1 includes the healthiest, lowest metabolic-load foods, such as fruits, whole oats, skinless meats, salmon, and fresh (not cooked) vegetables, and water. Zone 5 comprises the worst, highest-metabolic-load foods, such as pastries, donuts, chips, hard alcohol, high-fructose corn syrup, and deep fried foods, and sodas. You may notice that

a food's glycemic index—how quickly the carbohydrates break down (simple sugars and processed grain foods are among the highest and worst)—affects zone placement. So does how food is prepared: from best (Zone 1) to worst (Zone 5) are raw, steamed, baked, microwaved, and fried.

Like the Heart Zones, each of the five Food Zones is color-coded, with the lowest zones in the calm, gentle shades of blue, green, and yellow. The highest metabolic-load zones are in the hot colors—orange to scarlet red.

It's easy: If you stick to the low-zone metabolically light foods in the cool-colored Zones 1, 2, 3, and 4 that are below threshold—whole, natural, nutrient-rich foods—you will optimize your energy and health and help you avoid Syndrome X (also called "metabolic syndrome," a combination of disorders that can include high BMI, high blood pressure, high triglycerides, etc., and that increases the risk of developing cardiovascular disease and diabetes), diabetes, or other metabolic and cardiovascular diseases.

If you are ever a guest in my house, you might be amused by the "colorful" conversations we have. Yes, we actually talk about the color or number zone in which we spent most of our nutrient intake that day. "I had a tough day and ate mostly in the orange zone," I might say. "It's a Zone 4 day for me, but I had a blue zone breakfast." I encourage you to start talking the same language as you learn the benefits of eating a low-metabolic-load diet.

GET TO KNOW THE ZONES AND THE THRESHOLD LINE

The one key concept behind the Food Zones: eat below the threshold line. A threshold, like a door, is a crossover point between two spaces. In the Food Zones Chart, above the white threshold line are least-healthy foods (the red zone), and below it are healthier foods (the blue-green-yellow zones).

Staying in the low- to below-threshold zones will not be easy for those most saturated in our above-threshold nutrient culture. But understanding what you're doing is a big step toward making healthy changes and improving your

ZONE NUMBER	ZONE NAME	FAT	CARBOHYDRATE	PROTEIN	BEVERAGES	CHOCOLATE	FIBER GRAMS PER DAY	GLYCEMIC INDEX	QUALITY
5c	TOXIC ZONE	trans fats; non-dairy creamer, stick margarine, hydrogenated oil	table sugar	high fat meats	alcohol	less than 10% cocoa	0	>80	AVOID
5b	UNHEALTHY ZONE	chemically modified Fats: saturated fat, beef, whole milk, bacon fat	fructose	canned meat, bacon	espresso, soda	white chocolate 10%–20% cocoa	1	>75	VERY POOR
5a	LESS HEALTHY ZONE	high-fat cheese	cookies, chips, white bread, white rice	lunch meat with nitrates	fruit juice drinks	milk chocolate 20%–30% cocoa	1	>70	POOR

THE THRESHOLD LINE

ZONE NUMBER	ZONE NAME	FAT	CARBOHYDRATE	PROTEIN	BEVERAGES	CHOCOLATE	FIBER GRAMS PER DAY	GLYCEMIC INDEX	QUALITY
4	HEALTHY ZONE	monosaturated fats, olives, olive oil, peanuts, peanut butter, almonds, cashews–salted/roasted, avocados	processed grains, cereal	extra lean chicken/beef	beer, wine, 100% fruit juice	dark chocolate 30%–40% cocoa	1–2	70	GOOD
3	MORE HEALTHY ZONE	polysaturated fats: safflower oil, sesameseeds, walnuts, salmon, flax seeds–salted/roasted	whole grains	lean cuts of meat	decaf coffee, soy milk	sweet dark chocolate 40%–50% cocoa	2–4	60	VERY GOOD
2	HEALTHIER ZONE	monounsaturated & polyunsaturated fats–unsalted/roasted	beans, seeds	eggs, beans, seeds	low/non-fat milk, herb tea	semisweet chocolate 50%–60% cocoa	4–5	50	EXCELLENT
1	HEALTHIEST ZONE	monounsaturated & polyunsaturated fats–raw	fresh fruit and vegetables	wild fish	water	bittersweet chocolate 60%–85% cocoa	> 5	< 50	SUPERB

Figure 12.1

life. Here is an overview to the column headings across the top of the Food Zones Chart:

- **Zone number:** Higher numbers = lower quality foods. Eat in the low number zones.
- **Zone name:** Describes what happens if you eat in that zone on a regular basis.
- **Fat:** Lists the different types of fat; the fats in the low zones are the highest quality.
- **Carbohydrates/bread:** Describes the types of grains that are in bread in order of quality.
- **Protein:** Lists meats and vegetables with the least fat or the best quality of protein.
- **Beverages:** Includes the best liquids, with water being the best.
- **Chocolate:** A fun column for chocoholics showing which chocolates are healthiest.
- **Fiber grams:** Roughage from highest quality to foods with little to no fiber in the 5c zone.
- **Glycemic index:** Ranks carbohydrate effects on blood glucose levels. Low glycemic index carbohydrates are best.
- **Cooking:** Ranks food preparation—the least amount of food altering is the best choice.
- **Quality:** A rank from Superb to Avoid at All Costs.

HOW TO RUN OFF BODY FAT FOR GOOD

Many runners are aware that even skinny bodies have an almost unlimited supply of fat. Training to burn fat for fuel spares our very limited supply of stored carbohydrates (i.e., blood glucose or muscle and liver glycogen) for when we need to pick up the pace—a final kick, a long chase-down, a tough hill-climb. The big question is: How do you actually burn more fat? And doesn't fat only burn at a very low pace or aerobic zone?

The answer to the latter question is "no." There is no "fat-burning zone," as you might have seen printed on aerobic machines at the gym; that's a common misconception that I'll elaborate on a little later. The key point here is this: your body, in motion or not, burns both fat and carbs

for fuel at every speed, at every heart rate, in every heart zone. But the ratio of carbs to fat and total amount of calories burned changes with your effort and zone. In fact, while higher speeds require more carbs, they also generally burn the most fat, as you'll soon see.

FAT-BURNING FACTOR 1: HOW HARD AND LONG YOU RUN

The following table, developed by Gail Butterfield, Ph.D., for the Gatorade Sports Institute, shows the percentages of fat, carbohydrates, and protein burned in different exercise zones. On the chart, find the two columns "Total Calories per Minute" and "Fat Calories per Minute." You'll see that the calories burned per minute (assuming a 150-pound [68 kg] fit person with 20 percent to 25 percent body fat) rises from 2, 4, 7, and 10 in Zones 1–4, then spikes to 15, 30, and 50 in Zones 5a, 5b, and 5c (keeping in mind that you can't run for very long at Zone 5 speeds). Interestingly, even though the *percentage* of calories from fat burned decreases while speeding up, *the amount of fat metabolized* per minute actually increases as you speed up through the zones. You can see (in the second column) that the percentage of fat burned drops by nearly half: 80 percent to 45 percent from Zones 1 to 4, and then radically falls to zero by Zone 5c, the top end of an all-out sprint. But before that anaerobic rapid falloff, it turns out that you were actually burning more total fat, as shown in the last column on the right.

For example, our 150-pound (68 kg) fit person running for thirty minutes in Zone 3 will burn 7 calories per minute, for a total of 210 calories. Because 55 percent of those calories are fat, the total number of fat calories burned is 115.5.

Those numbers jump if our runner speeds up to Zone 4. Although the percentage of fat burned drops to 45 percent, the total amount of fat, as well as calories overall, increases. The math: thirty minutes in Zone 4 burns 300 calories (10 calories per minute × 30), and 135 fat calories (300 × 45 percent). Bottom line: Zone 4 burns 90 more total calories and 20.5 more fat calories than Zone 3. Similarly pronounced differences also occur while comparing Zone 1 and Zone 2 to Zone 3 and Zone 4.

ZONE #	% OF FAT CALORIES BURNED	% OF CARB CALORIES BURNED	% OF PROTEIN CALORIES BURNED	TOTAL CAL./MIN.	FAT CAL./MIN.
Zone 1	80%	15%	5%	2	1.6
Zone 2	75%	20%	5%	4	3.0
Zone 3	55%	40%	5%	7	3.85
Zone 4	45%	50%	5%	10	4.5
Zone 5a	20%	75%	5%	15	3.0
Zone 5b	10%	85%	5%	30	3.0
Zone 5c	0%	95%	5%	50	0

This example illustrates the fallacy of the illusionary, super-slow fat-burning zone that you might find on a chart imprinted on your treadmill. Notice that fat burning isn't one of the five threshold zones—because there is no one, single fat-burning zone! Every zone, except for the last all-out sliver of Zone 5, burns fat. The concept of a single fat-burning zone, invented by coaches and fitness professionals in an attempt to simplify the concept of calorie burning, has led to a great deal of confusion about how fat is utilized when you run.

In reality, there is quite a wide fat-burning range that extends all the way to your threshold. From Zones 1 through 4, you burn both fat and carbs for fuel. As you cross the threshold into Zone 5, however, you actually start going too fast to burn a significant amount of fat. Here's why. On a technical level, it's all about oxygen. Working muscle cells require the presence of oxygen to burn fat as a source of fuel. That means that faster, anaerobic speeds burn smaller percentages of fat. When you run above your threshold intensity (T_1), the crossover point between sustainable and nonsustainable running pace, you burn little fat, and you burn zero fat above the second threshold point (T_2), which is basically an all-out sprint that you can maintain for only a few seconds.

The bottom line is that to burn the most fat in the least amount of time, you must run briskly while staying aerobic, which means keeping below threshold—staying out of Zone 5—and spending as much time as possible in Zone 4.

But that doesn't mean you shouldn't push yourself to go faster. Here's why.

FAT-BURNING FACTOR 2: HOW FIT YOU ARE

Besides upgrading your *quantity* of running in Zone 4 to burn more fat and total calories, you can also burn more by upgrading the *quality* of your Zone 4. That means raising Zone 4 to a higher threshold heart rate. You do this by getting fitter.

Significant fat burning starts where aerobic benefits are first measured, at about 60 percent of threshold (T_1). As you get fitter, your T_1 moves upward toward your maximum heart rate, and your fat-burning range gets bigger. So, if you want to lose more weight, make it your goal to get fitter and raise your T_1, which will expand your fat-burning range.

How do you do it? Training above the fat-burning range once or twice per week for two or three months, using intervals and fast tempo runs, will push up your threshold.

BREAK THE DIET-AND-GET-FATTER CYCLE

"One might wonder whether dieting has been one of the major causes of obesity," somewhat cynically writes my dear friend and colleague from Australia, Dr. David Richards, M.D., in his wonderful book *Being Alive*. There are infinite causes of weight gain, more weight-loss diets than ever, and few long-term solutions. Like Dr. Richards said, the more we diet the fatter we seem to get.

Losing long-term weight is one of the most challenging goals to accomplish, with or without medical supervision. The failure rate is above 95 percent. Why can't people, even many runners, lose weight? One of the reasons is the myth that the laws of thermodynamics work consistently in humans.

The laws of thermodynamics say that calories in equal calories out (or CI = CO). But while the so-called energy-balancing equation means the calories you eat equal the calories you expend, it is unfortunately not the case, and several examples will show why.

One example is menopause, when many women suddenly gain weight, despite no change in diet or lifestyle. The reason? A change in hormones.

Another example is a recent study in which 35,000 people took a low-dose vitamin D pill (which has zero calories) and lost more weight than those who took the placebo. Vitamin D, which modern humans chronically lack, helps you lose weight because it is important for metabolic processing. But again, it has no calories, proving the CI = CO formula invalid—and proving that something else is happening: metabolic fitness.

METABOLIC FITNESS: YOUR BEST METABOLISM

Metabolism is defined as the summation of all the vital energy-requiring processes (heart beat, breathing, digestion, and other bodily functions), chemical reactions, and activities (from running to driving a car or shopping) that occur in the course of your day and life. Metabolism is like your car engine at idle, revving away. The faster your metabolism, the more energy you need, calories you burn, and weight you lose. The slower your metabolism, the harder it is to get the pounds off.

Scientists report that the speed of your metabolism is stable and can't be changed from its basic rate, although it can be revved up regularly for limited time periods. Some believe a faster metabolism can be achieved if you:

- **Add muscle.** Bigger muscles need more calories to work than smaller muscles.
- **Exercise often.** Metabolic rate rises during and immediately after exercise, and after a hard interval or weight workout, it stays higher longer.
- **Eat regular meals.** There is a thermic effect of eating—yes, the act of eating burns calories, so eat every three to four hours to keep the fires burning. Don't skip meals—it signals the body to slow down and save fat.
- **Eat longer meals.** People consume more calories when they wolf down food. You get more hormones that produce feelings of satiety when you eat slowly.
- **Stay hydrated.** Thirst and hunger are often confused; drink more water and you'll eat less.
- **Stay cooler.** Colder weather revs up the metabolism in order to keep the body warmer.

A well-functioning metabolism not only metabolizes fat efficiently, but also protects you from unpleasant health conditions. "Being metabolically fit means having a metabolism that maximizes vitality and minimizes the risk of disease—particularly those diseases that are influenced by lifestyle, such as heart disease, type 2 diabetes, and cancer," says Glenn A. Gaesser, Ph.D., at Arizona State University and the author of a book that I love, *Big Fat Lies*. Revealing how well or efficiently your metabolism works, metabolic fitness is a relatively new piece of the running-for-fitness puzzle that you can measure in several ways, including assessing your insulin resistance and sensitivity (blood sugar levels), resting and exercise metabolic rates, blood pressure, and cholesterol levels.

REAL WEIGHT-LOSS TIPS FROM PEOPLE WHO HAVE KEPT IT OFF

Every year, millions of new diet books are sold in the United States. One of the best answers to long-term weight loss can be found in the example of those who have *maintained* their weight loss. These *applied* weight-loss experts have discovered what works for their physiology, genetics, and emotional nature. You'll hear about their revelations a little later in the chapter.

One of the worst effects of weight cycling (repeated weight loss and gain) is the redistribution of body fat to the upper compartments of your abdomen. This abdominal (or visceral) fat resides in and around your organs, and has been strongly associated with chronic high-risk diseases. If that isn't bad enough, weight cycling also leads to a reduction in metabolic rates known as "adaptive thermogenesis." Basically, the more often you weight cycle, the lower your resting metabolic rate, or your base caloric burn rate, becomes.

Where's the hope in all this bad news? Well, that's where those applied weight-loss experts come in. The National Weight Control Registry (www.nwcr.ws) is a nonprofit organization that tracks people who have kept more than thirty pounds (13.6 kg) of weight off for more than one year. Of the 5,000-plus Americans that they follow (80 percent are women, 20 percent men), the average woman is forty-five and weights 145 pounds (66 kg), while the average man is forty-nine and weighs 190 pounds (86 kg). Participants' losses ranged from thirty pounds (13.6 kg) to 300 pounds (136 kg). While some lost weight rapidly and others slowly, over as many as fourteen years, nearly all did it through a hard working focus on both diet *and* exercise:

- Some lost it on their own (45 percent) and others followed a dietary program (55 percent).
- Ninety-eight percent of participants reported that they modified their food intake.
- Ninety-four percent increased their physical activity, with walking the most popular activity.

The three keys to what The National Weight Control Registry members (and they are looking for new members—you can register on their website) report for weight maintenance are: low calorie consumption, low fat in their diet, and a high level of daily physical activity. For example:

- 78 percent eat breakfast every day.
- 75 percent weigh themselves at least once a week.
- 62 percent watch fewer than ten hours of TV per week.
- 90 percent exercise an average of one hour per day.

So, while each runner must find what works for his or her individual metabolism and genetic makeup, we can all thank these women and men for discovering some common denominators in losing weight and keeping it off. You would be wise to follow the lead of the few and the successful. Ultimately, I believe each of us must take responsibility for our own weight gain or loss.

ADDITIONAL DIETING TIPS

Everybody responds to food differently—no single diet plan fits everyone—and expecting anyone to stick 100-percent to any plan is unrealistic. However, I believe that by following a few diet guidelines, everyone can simplify the challenge of eating for enhanced running. Here are a few that I follow:

- **Remember the rule of three times.** Eat three times the fruits and vegetables as you do meat and fat.
- **Keep a balance.** Each meal should contain the three food groups: carbohydrates, protein, and fat.
- **Go for good emotional foods.** Comfort foods and food cravings are normal. Try to respond by choosing foods in the lower Food Zones.
- **Convert your tribe.** Surround yourself with those who also eat a good, cardio-metabolic diet. Encourage your entire family to eat from the Food Zones Chart and to eat in the blue-green-yellow zones.
- **Eat in or take it to go.** To better control portion sizes and nutrient density, and to ingest fewer processed foods, eating in or packing a meal-to-go is your best choice.

- **Mind your Qs.** It is better to eat less quantity but more quality.
- **Think nutrient-dense.** Frequently eat small amounts of whole foods packed with nutrients.
- **Eat to lighten your load.** Eat to fuel your workouts and your life, but eat nutritious foods that have low metabolic load.
- **Eat low-GI foods.** Not all carbohydrates are equal; eat those with a low glycemic index.
- **Cheat occasionally.** It's not essential to eat exclusively in the four low zones—what you do *most of the time* is what matters. Exceptions are permitted—it's only human nature. Just don't do it too much.
- **This is not a diet, but a lifestyle.** Think of low-zone eating as the way you should eat all the time, not as a diet for a certain period of time.
- **Eat high-energy foods.** Eat lots of fruit, vegetables, whole grains, fish, and lean meats.
- **Drink and be merry.** Drink lots of fluids, preferably water and below-threshold fluids.
- **During heavy training, eat more calorie-dense foods.** To get more fuel in the tank in periods of big miles, eat more cheese, nuts, avocados, beans, peanut butter on wheat bread, whole milk, and salad dressing.
- **Try new stuff.** Continually add a variety of healthy foods to your diet to keep it interesting and exciting.

HYDRATION

From experience, we all know that running in the heat is more difficult than training or racing in moderate conditions. This is due to environmental heat stress. The other source of heat stress while running is mechanical heat. As you run faster your body heats up from the increased metabolic output from muscle contractions (thermogenesis). Without care and proper hydration, thermogenesis can lead to heatstroke, fatigue, and overheating.

In 1994 I entered the first Eco Challenge Adventure Race in southeast Utah's canyon lands. The Eco Challenge is a coed team event; I raced with a team of four experienced athletes including a mountain bike champ, an ultra-marathoner, a white water raft guide, a physician and myself—four men and one woman. There were seven different events in the race, which was a continuously timed, start-to-finish race leaving little time to sleep during the 10 days required to complete the 350 mile (563 km) course. Since the course was kept secret prior to race day, no one could test the availability of water. For our water supply, we decided to depend on the ample supply of wells marked on our map of the area.

The first of the seven events was a 25-mile (40 km) ride-and-run with three horses per team. With five team members, we alternated riding and running, three riding and two running at any given time. We finished the first event in third place out of 55 teams and were then given maps for the next event: a 110-mile (177 km) run. The first fifty miles (80.5 km) snaked through narrow slot canyons, where we were repeatedly plunging into deep and frigid water, still wearing our backpacks. After finishing the slot canyon section, we began the final 60 miles (96.5 km), which we called the Bataan Death March. During World War II, after the Battle of Bataan, a forced march of 60 miles (96.5 km) in the jungle heat with almost no water resulted in the death of hundreds or even thousands of POWs from heat stroke. We imagined this would be our fate, too, when we discovered that the wells on our map were dry. The one well containing water was contaminated, a dead cow floating there ominously. As the helicopters flew in to evacuate other teams, we grimly realized that we had to ration our water to survive to the end of the stage. Tongues swollen, lips cracked, and the pace slowed from the fatiguing effects of dehydration, we finished the event, barely.

Staying properly hydrated is vital to your running success, but it is more about heat than about drinking fluids. Sure, you have to replace the fluid loss, but your principal goal is to manage heat stress, which can be a killer. The key is to manage your body's core temperature while avoiding dehydration. Drinking too much water, thereby reducing the ratio of necessary salts, can result in a condition called hyponatremia, which can be just as deadly—if not more so—as dehydration. Staying sufficiently hydrated is a balance of competing mechanisms. Drinking too much fluid results in what Timothy Noakes describes in *The Lore of Running* as "overdrinking phenomenon" or water intoxication. Excessive drinking often occurs on long runs over several hours, typically at low velocity with high hydration. It's a bit complicated, but basically when you over drink, your stomach needs salts to dissolve the sodium ions in the intestines. The salt, sodium and chloride ions provided by the bloodstream to the intestines reduces the salts' concentration in the blood. Sodium concentration in the blood lowers and hyponatremia develops. A runner experiencing hyponatremia becomes disoriented and, if severe, can suffer serious brain function disturbances and possible brain oedema, which can be severe enough to be fatal.

One of the principal mechanisms to regulate temperature while running is sweating. Glands in the skin produce fluid that evaporates, causing heat to be transferred away from the body via convection. As body core temperature increases, normal cardiac response increases blood flow to the skin and away from the non-working muscles in order to cool internal systems, including the working muscles, by the mechanism of sweating. A slow increase in heart rate, called "cardiac drift," accompanies any increase in core temperature. Cardiac drift is normal and is a direct result of two different thermo regulation response outcomes: dehydration and core temperature rising.

As you become dehydrated, your plasma volume drops (blood thickening or haemo-concentration) and your cardiac output—how much blood is pumped with each heartbeat—drops from insufficient blood volume, causing your heart rate to increase or drift upward. It is difficult while running to assess the cause of increasing heart rate when pace is maintained, but heart rate is slowly sliding upward toward the next zone—a place you prefer not to go when focusing on steady-state pacing. Are the heart rate numbers escalating because of dehydration, meaning you need to drink

more or differently? Or are they escalating because core body temperature increases are causing blood to be preferentially directed to the skin for cooling, meaning you should attempt to cool off by pouring water over your head or mopping your skin with a sponge?

Cardiac drift is one good reason to use a heart rate monitor. This response to environmental and cardiovascular load from heat resulting in heart rate increases makes it especially important to use your heart rate monitor when you are running in the heat to monitor these responses. And a speed-and-distance monitor is useful to determine if you are increasing or decreasing your speed. Training tools like these can help you make smart, cognitive decisions based on accurate biofeedback information before, during, or after running.

In hot conditions, you can't absorb fluids fast enough to replace the fluid losses from sweating. This is why maintaining your hydration during high intensity competition is nearly impossible. Drinking more isn't the problem because at high intensity, the absorption rate of fluid is slower than the demand for it. In a stressful thermal environment, the fluid loss via sweat is simply greater than your ability to compensate by drinking. When the temperatures climb above 85°F (over 30°C), your sweat rate is about 34 to 85 fluid ounces (1000-2500 ml) per hour. Meanwhile, your ability to absorb fluid during high intensity exercise is reduced because blood is shunted away from the stomach and intestines—lowering absorption rates—to the skin in order to enhance sweat rate to reduce core temperature. The peak fluid absorption per hour during running for the average sized runner is 24 fluid ounces (700 ml). Do the math; no matter how you try to balance the numbers, you cannot overcome the fact that, while exercising hard in the heat, you sweat faster than you can absorb fluids.

When competing, a key reason to avoid dehydration is not the immediate health risks but premature fatigue. Premature fatigue, the first feeling of the inability to maintain your pace, happens for most runners upon losing about 7%-10% of their body weight. When reaching this level of dehydration, blood pressure drops, heart rate and core temperature increase, the heart's output and stroke volume decrease, and blood flow to the skin decreases. These physiological changes are all in proportion to the degree of dehydration: it is a linear reaction. However, you can recover rapidly and can return to performance within minutes by drinking and lying down to rest. Health risks arise if you become dehydrated beyond 15%-20% of body weight. Beyond 20% body weight loss, there is the risk of death. Always drink sufficiently to stay below the 15% threshold.

Trying to force yourself to drink at rates equal to rates of sweat loss just does not work well. Research and my own experience agree that drinking voluntarily during running is just as beneficial as forcing myself to drink fluids based on specific amounts at specific time periods. If I try to force myself to drink to match sweat rates and body weight loss, I usually wind up feeling bloated. It is important to drink voluntarily at rates approaching or slightly lower than your sweat rate to avoid the physiological disturbances that result in premature fatigue.

Drinking too much fluid high in calories (sugars) or that is too cold can result in stomach cramps. Race directors cannot be expected to mix the fluids at aid stations in the right proportions for you (or to provide sanitary drinking conditions). Not all commercially available drinks meet a runner's physiological requirements or are sufficiently digestible for every runner. If you have a sensitive stomach, you need to know what will work for you before the race and make your own plans if what is provided is not on your list of "good" hydration choices.

Many runners drink large volumes of water long before a race, practicing a ritual of hyperhydration. Hyperhydration is one of those running myths that just isn't substantiated by research. Humans are different from camels and cannot store large amounts of water. Drinking such amounts of fluids before a big training run or a race; rather than preventing dehydration, simply results in frequent bathroom stops.

THE OPTIMUM SPORTS DRINK

In 1978, I entered the first 75-mile (121 km) around Lake Tahoe Run. Having only finished a half dozen marathons and one 50 mile (80.5 km) race prior to that, I had almost no experience at ultra running. Back then, there were few ultra runners on the planet to query about how often and what to drink. The only sports drink on the market at the time was Gookinaid, developed by San Diego chemist, Bill Gookin. Taking his lead, I suspected that there must be a way to get nutrients—calories and electrolytes—from my gut into my blood stream, sparing my stored glucose levels and my liver from having to serve up carbohydrates that I might need down-the-road.

So I went into the kitchen with my secret list of ingredients that I thought would help me perform: aspirin for pain (there was no ibuprofen), bee pollen (I don't know why), sugar from Coke for energy, table salt to replace the sodium that working muscles need, and water to dilute the ingredients, because I suspected that my stomach would revolt if I didn't dilute the recipe. I tested this formula in advance on a training run at sea level on a cool day, and it worked perfectly. I felt that I had more energy and that my gut was comfortable—little did I know what would happen when fatigue, altitude, heat, and stress combined together to wreak havoc.

On the day of the race, temperatures soared. Lake Tahoe, at an altitude of over 6,000 feet (1,828 m), can cause most runners some altitude distress. I followed the old rule of the time to drink on a timeline and a fixed amount rather than drinking freely. And I decided to drink as much as I possibly could. At 30 miles (48 km) into the race, in the high heat of the day, I developed a distended and swollen stomach with a sphincter valve that slammed closed, preventing the absorption of my special aspirin-bee's pollen-salt-sugar filled energy drink concoction. Fortunately, my Shiatsu expert and friend Steve Tamaribuchi (now famous for the development of his eGrip training devices) was on my support team. After I slowed, complaining about the gastric pain, Steve gently applied pressure on a spot near my sternum, and I felt a relieving gush as the valve magically opened and the stopped-up fluids in my stomach drained quickly into my small intestines. My swollen belly shrank, my legs picked up the pace again, and I finished second, completing the 75-mile (121 km) course in 13 hours.

That was over 30 years ago, and exercise science researchers have since replaced guessing with research showing what runners really need in an ideal sports drink. Today, a lot more is known about the need for intestinal absorption of carbohydrates, electrolyte replacements, the gastric emptying rates of fluids, variations in palatability, and, our individual physiology. Whether purchased commercially or a formula of your own created in the kitchen, the consensus of scientists is as follows:

- Sodium concentration of 20-60 mmol per liter of fluid.
- Carbohydrate concentration of 7.5%-12% depending on the rate at which you are drinking.
- Mixed carbohydrates such as glucose and maltodextrins to keep a low to moderate osmolality and for taste.

The old adage to drink often and as much as possible has not held up against both lab and practical tests. Over-drinking does not prevent the adverse effects of heat and fatigue because the effects of mechanical heat and environmental heat cannot always be compensated by your rate of fluid absorption. Proper hydration with the right balance of fluid, energy, and electrolytes is a delicate balance depending on running speed, elapsed running time, environmental conditions, and your own genetic propensity to heat tolerance and ability to stay hydrated. You should try to drink fluids at approximately the same rate you are using them, but realize particularly in the heat, this may not be feasible. Conversely, it can be detrimental to your performance to drink excessively in extreme heat. My approach is to drink, according to thirst and approximate sweat rate, fluids that best maintain my hydration, while still contributing to sodium and carbohydrate levels.

HYDRATION TIPS

Here are a few quick tips to help you stay hydrated and manage your fluid intake:

1. Weight. Weigh yourself daily to assess your hydration. A reduction in over 4% of body weight may indicate fluid deficiency. Drink more to reduce this hydration stress.

2. Thirst. Drink before you are thirsty: often, by the time you are thirsty, you are already 5% or more dehydrated.

3. Pre-Run. Drink before your workout and again about every 20-30 minutes in warmer weather.

4. Post Run. Continue hydrating as soon as possible after every workout.

5. Over 60 Minute Rule. If you are running for more than 60 minutes, drink electrolyte solutions with a 5%-8% carbohydrate mixture.

6. High Temperatures. Always modify your workout when the temperatures soar. If over 85°F (over 30°C), limit the duration of your run to prevent heat stress: run short, run in the shade, run carrying water. A good rule of thumb is to reduce everything to 75% or below: speed, zone, and effort.

7. Greatest Fluid Loss. Longer and more intensive workouts—the high training zones—cause the most dehydration.

8. Sports Drinks. Test them in training runs. The digestibility of sports drinks varies considerably between runners, hence the proliferation of products and theories about which ones work the best and the fastest.

9. Delay. Delay heat exposure and therefore hydration demands before the start of a race or training by staying in an air-conditioned room, using ice treatments, and staying wet to defer the effects of heat stress.

10. Racing. Cool off during a race by using wet sponges on your skin or pouring water over your head. Ice packs around the neck are also a convenient way to lower blood temperature.

11. Two Hours and Two Minutes Before the Race. Stop drinking about two hours before the race to allow enough time to empty your bladder. For any race longer than a 10K, about two minutes before the race, drink again about 400-500 ml of fluids.

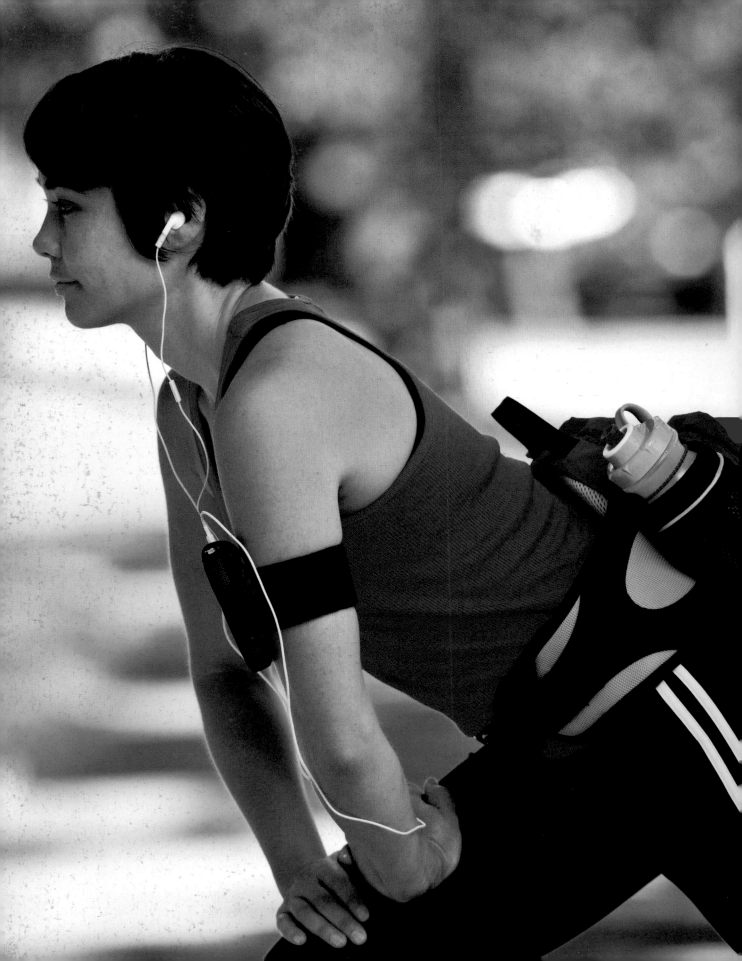

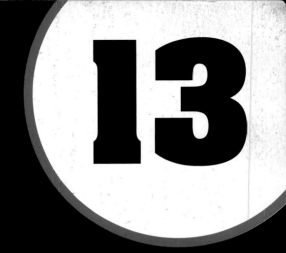

SAFETY FOR ALL TYPES OF RUNNERS: RUNNING WITHOUT RISK

ONE OF MY FREQUENT RUNNING PARTNERS IS ADI ADI, my 40-pound (18 kg) Australian shepherd mutt, eleven years old as I write this in 2010. I found her at the pound and it was love at first sight. One winter day when I was in my late fifties, I took up a new sport extreme sledding— and she joined me. She herds cows and sleds at our rustic cabin in the Sierra Nevadas. Bringing her along turned out to be a smart move, because on my first trip down the advanced hill, I crashed and broke my back.

Barely able to move and in excruciating pain, I looked at Adi Adi and said, "Go home, girl." She ran off and I fought not to pass out. Thirty minutes later, my cell phone—which I'd forgotten about in my fanny pack—rang. "She's home, but you're not." said my partner. "What happened?"

I'm not the first one to have her life saved by a dog. In a horrific incident in 2006, superstar ultra-runner/adventure racer Danelle Ballangee slipped while out for a two-hour "easy jog" with her dog Taz on a remote, icy cliff a few miles outside her home in Moab, Utah. She fell 60 feet (97 km) down a rock ledge, shattered her pelvis and sacrum, splattered her internal organs, and lay helpless through two freezing nights. Close to death on the third day, she was saved when Taz, a brown German shepherd/golden retriever mix, was found wandering and led rescuers to the scene.

Having a dog along as you are getting in your running (or hiking/snowshoeing/sledding) workout is one of many safety and motivational tools that is often overlooked. For most runners, safety usually starts and ends with reflective clothing. But there's a lot more to this not-so-prosaic topic than that. You literally run a risk every time you go out for a jog. Cars, predators, illnesses, and injuries are lurking nearby, ready to strike. To stay safe, you need a plan.

This chapter discusses lots of gear and strategies to keep all types of runners—beginners, women, older athletes, and even strapping, virile men—out of harm's way. And, of course, not least among them is a canine companion—I've had four of them in the past forty years—who can add safety and joy to your running in ways you may not have ever imagined.

ADVICE FOR ALL RUNNERS

Figuring out how to avoid unfriendly fellow travelers on the roads and trails—from ill-intentioned animals and humans to faceless metal objects outweighing them by 4,000 pounds (1,814 kg)—is a runner's primary concern.

SAFETY AND SURVIVAL TIPS

Accordingly, the most basic runners' safety and survival tips focus on runners seeing and being seen and, if necessary, keeping in touch with the love ones back home.

- **Don't expect cars and bikes to see you.** Be extra careful at cross streets. Don't think vehicles see you as you cross the street or run parallel to them. They don't.
- **Wear bright clothes.** To be seen and avoided by cars, do not put fashion first—unless it's colored fluorescent yellow, orange, and green. The more garish the better.
- **Wear a reflective running vest and other gear at night.** Don't be invisible when lighting is insufficient, such as after dark, in the early morning, and in inclement weather. Purchase reflective patches, too, affixing them to your shoes and hat. Car drivers will see you when your torso lights up from a half-mile away.
- **Run against traffic and carry ID.** You need to see them before they hit you. If you can see an oncoming obstacle, you can try to avoid it. Five years ago, a guy in Grass Valley, California, running with (not against) traffic, was hit in the back of the head by the huge traffic mirror of a truck and was instantly killed. It took the authorities three days to identify him. Have a wrist bracelet with your ID on it or carry a business card in your fanny pack.

- **Take the road less traveled.** Running on less-crowded back roads and nonmotorized paths exposes you to fewer cars and exhaust. But watch out for bikes.
- **Tell someone.** Before you take off on a run, give your loved ones some idea of the route you'll be running. That will let them at least have someplace to start looking for you if they get worried.
- **Beware of mountain lions (and other wild animals) on the trail.** Off-road running is a joy and is far easier on your knees than pounding pavement, but the danger posed by mountain lions is real in mountainous areas, such as where I live in California. Attacks are rare but more frequent with the encroachment of civilization on the natural habitat. In 1994, an acquaintance of mine, Barbara Schoener, 5' 11" (180 cm) tall, 140 pounds (64 kg), ran alone one day on the Western States 100 trail near Auburn and didn't come back. A mountain lion had ambushed her, killed her, dragged her off the trail, and buried her. The next day, the rangers caught and killed the lion. Turns out it was a lactating mother with a cub, which was then put in the local Folsom, California, zoo. The mountain lion was doing what is natural—protecting her cubs when threatened. I have also seen rattlesnakes and, believe it or not, surprisingly aggressive turkeys on the trail. The bottom line is that the trail poses its own risks. Therefore:
- **Run with a companion—human or canine.** The excitement, camaraderie, and routine of running with other people on both road and trail are great motivation and supply you with a built-in bodyguard. Dogs, who love the attention and exercise, serve the same purpose. Their very presence forces other creatures—two- or four-legged—to keep their distance.
- **Carry a cell phone and ID in your fanny pack.** It'll come in handy when you're kidnapped, knocked into a ditch, or merely too tired to run those 12 miles (19 km) back home. Preparing for a worst-case scenario costs little and can save your life.

- **Be ready to turn tail.** If something threatening lurks ahead—gang members, a traffic accident, stray dogs, arrogant horseback riders—swallow your pride and turn right around.
- **Become a student of running.** Reading the magazines will give you valuable tips about races, gear, and safety issues, and get you familiar with the legends of the sport. This active information gathering will give you more of a stake in running and something to talk about with your partners, who in turn provide the safety of a group.
- **Join a group.** Do it for the camaraderie, the fitness, and the local knowledge about good places to run and races. The commitment to run with others is fun and motivating, and will keep you running more.
- **Rest a cold.** There has long been a debate about the risk of running through a runny nose. While there is no conclusive proof that bed rest cures a respiratory virus any faster, my recommendation is to take it easy. That means no more than a light jog with a minor cold, and no workout at all beyond that—especially with a fever. Your heart is already working double time by maintaining metabolic function and pumping blood to the skin's surface to reduce the fever's heat. Don't add a third load onto your system.

FIGHTING OVERUSE INJURIES

Put stress on muscles and they get stronger. Put too much stress on muscles for too long and they fatigue and put the body at risk for illness.

We've known for a long while now that the most common running injuries are caused by a single culprit: overuse. Overuse injuries generally fall into two categories: stress fractures and inflammation of the tendons, ligaments, bursa, cartilage, connective tissues, or nerve tissues.

These overuse injuries are caused by repeated stress and trauma on a given structure in training, which overwhelms its capacity to respond and repair itself.

Overtraining is almost entirely due to excessive mileage, with a strong contribution from the too-much or too-soon category, such as the following:
- Too fast an increase in the distances in your training schedule
- Too much of an increase in resistance training, such as climbing hills
- Too much interval training, too soon
- Too many or too intense bounding or jumping exercises
- Too much time spent running on hard surfaces

Other injuries are caused by training errors, such as the wrong shoes, inadequate stretching/warming up, inadequate flexibility and/or strength, imbalanced muscle development, and uncompensated leg-length differences.

For overuse injuries, rest is the best treatment. However, if your condition is serious, casting, crutches, anti-inflammatory drugs, or physical therapy may be required. For less serious injuries, it's permissible to treat it yourself first by using the RICE formula: rest, ice, compression, and elevation of the injured part.

If you have continued or chronic pain, get a diagnosis and treatment. You can't keep the problem from recurring if you don't know its cause. Every overuse injury is caused by a force on a tissue that is greater than the tissue's basic strength, and every injury-causing force can be traced to one of the following causes:
- Training errors that do not allow for adequate recovery
- Tissues that are weak and susceptible to injury
- Biomechanical weaknesses that put excessive stress on certain parts of your body

When you know what caused pain, you can begin to fix it.

Rehabilitation, using flexibility, strengthening, and aerobic/high-intensity conditioning, is the key to returning to your training program. If you are injured, cross-train in a different skill that doesn't hurt, until the pain disappears. If you continue to train with pain, you only exacerbate the problem and delay healing.

PREVENTING MINOR TRAINING INJURIES

Minor discomforts are your body's way of telling you that something is out of balance, ill-fitting, or overstressed. Ignore them too long and they might flare into larger problems. Here's how to handle the most common ones:

- **Blisters**—lube liberally. Blisters are inevitable for feet, underarms, and men's nipples (see the "Advice for Men" section, page 199). The last couple miles of running with unlubed blisters can be excruciating and potentially put you out of commission for several days. Lube up before and, if necessary, during the run to minimize the damage. You can deal with foot blisters, often caused by ill-fitting shoes that have tight spots, by using a medicated cream and bandage if the blister is small; drain the blister first if it is large.

- **Black toenails**—wear looser shoes. This condition is caused by pounding your toes against the inside of the front of the shoe, which typically occurs during downhills. You can avoid it by wearing shoes half a size larger than your regular shoe.

- **Tripping**—use lace locks and elastic shoe laces. The fact is that you will trip. Don't assume that you're a klutz or incompetent; it happens to everyone—on uneven, root-studded trails and even on perfectly smooth pavement. It seems like I trip once a year. But you can and should reduce the chance of tripping on untied laces and getting some part of your body bloody by using lace locks. They're dirt-cheap and convenient, so there's no excuse for not using them.

 Once Trained, Women Do Not Get Injured More

- **Trail tumbles**—wear gloves. You will certainly trip occasionally on the rocks, holes, and debris on dirt trails, so take a cue from mountain bikers and protect your hands.
- **Muscle cramps**—seek help with a variety of solutions. Knot-like, involuntary muscle contractions indicate something is out of whack—you could be dehydrated or low on sodium, potassium, calcium, and various vitamins. To get home from your run, hydrate, stretch, massage, walk it off, and resume running at a gradual pace. Walk if running is too painful—or use that cell phone. If cramps persist, try a new diet and fluid plan.
- **Side stitch**—rub it out. Thought to be caused by over-exertion and gas in the large intestine, a side stitch can be handled with this self-massage: Put your fingers on the sore spot and apply pressure. Massage the entire area with your whole hand, straighten your back and stretch tall, relax your breathing, and slow the number of breaths you take per minutes, lean forward, and bend at the waist.
- **Nausea**—time your eating. Don't eat right before the workout. Not only will the calories not have time to be utilized for the workout, but it'll upset your stomach. Dehydration exacerbates the problem.

ADVICE FOR OLDER RUNNERS

Age takes a toll on everyone over the age of forty, changing the bodies and needs of middle-aged runners. To stay safe in that demographic, follow all the rules in the rest of this chapter and add these:

- **Do strength-speed exercises to regain your quick-reaction time.** Quickness slows with age, making it harder to respond to imbalances and prevent falls. But you can mitigate this effect somewhat by doing plyometrics and rapid-contraction weight training.
- **Cross-train more.** All my friends over age fifty say they need more recovery time from running. To get it, but not get out of aerobic shape, hit the pool, the bike, the elliptical machine, the rower, and anything that pushes your heart rate but rests your running-specific muscles.

- **Run with younger people.** Your fitness can suffer if your aging peer group slows your pace below your ability, or if they don't show up at all—an increasingly common occurrence with an older crowd. That's why, when I was pushing sixty, I began running with my high-energy friend Pam, who's twenty-eight. She runs a little faster than I like—but I don't tell her. I met Pam by joining a club called the Pink House, which is held in a home in my neighborhood that holds daily spinning classes in its garage. Like most younger people, she's more into technology than my age group, so I have a lot of fun chatting and comparing notes with her about the latest computers, heart rate monitors, and speed and distance gizmos.
- **Do longer warm-ups.** While I've generally never done much of a warm-up, I've started rethinking that. The evidence is pretty clear that lungs and muscles are slower to initially respond to exercise and joints are slower to bath themselves in synovial fluids. A long, gradual warm-up will help you avoid muscle strain and joint pain.
- **Stretch more.** Since muscles lose elasticity as you age, stretching is increasingly important. Check Chapter 5 for details on when and what stretches to do.

ADVICE FOR WOMEN

Women have two challenges: staying safe while training and dealing with unique physical health issues. The following two sections describe both.

SAFETY ON THE ROADS

In today's society, unfortunately, it can be dangerous for a woman to run alone. The risk of being a victim of a crime is very real. Therefore, the major concerns of women runners, beyond the previous tips common to all runners, start with reducing any potential threat from aggressive males and the opportunity for being a target:

- **Run a different route every day.** Habitually running in the same place at the same time every day is easy on your schedule, but also makes it easy for assailants to plan an attack. Vary your patterns so that no one can lay in wait for you.

- **Don't run at night.** The risk is multiplied when assailants are cloaked in darkness. If you must run at night, run in open, well-lit areas.
- **Don't wear expensive jewelry, lots of makeup, and revealing clothing.** Be smart and ditch your vanity; don't call attention to yourself or give anyone a reason to try to be attracted to you. The fewer valuables on you, and the more modest your clothing, the less likely you'll be hassled.
- **Pack a fight-back tool.** Carry a whistle, a can of mace, pepper spray, or any deterrent you can use as a weapon and as a way to get bystanders' attention.
- **Run with a partner, human or canine.** I already said this is what every runner should do, but it's worth reemphasizing for women: Don't travel alone. You're safest with another body running at your side. One man can overpower a woman, but not two women.
- **Also, a buddy comes in handy when you hurt yourself: For example, I once tripped while running and broke my ankle.** The damage from walking home and dragging my foot caused months of delay in my recovery and left me an easy target.
- **And regarding dogs: Everyone respects you and keeps their distance when you have Fido along.** Use a leash when you run in the city. Let the dog loose (when it is legal to do so) on the trails, but train him to stay with you. That maintains your protection but lets you focus more on the irregular terrain.
- **Know your turf.** Get familiar with your running routes, even to the point of getting to know some of the residents along the way. Know where there is dense foliage or other spots in which assailants can hide. Don't get trapped in areas that you can't find your way out of or your way home from. Here's another hint: Put an energy bar and dog biscuit in your fanny pack (along with the standard cell phone and ID). The shortest run can be an adventure, so be prepared. The human and doggie treats are for those runner's-high rambles when you got lost or you got carried away and ran an hour extra.

- **Be alert, don't space out, and turn down the music.** Never trust that you are perfectly safe—because you aren't. Blocking out your senses with headphones while enjoyable and motivating, is risky. It's vital for your safety that you see and hear what's going on around you.
- **Have a plan to flee, fight, and scream.** Remind yourself that it's dangerous out there, that even a seemingly safe route can turn risky in an instant. Therefore, make a plan for what you'll do when a person enters your personal-space safety zone. Be ready to scream, run away to areas with people, and if you have to, fight back (if the assailant is unarmed). Claw at the face and the eyes, shout at the top of your lungs, be heard and seen, create a disturbance, and make a scene. Yell "Fire!" or "Police!" Use profanity if you have to; it's worth it if it keeps you alive. Also, have some self-defense skills.
- **Take a self-defense class.** A martial arts/self-defense class specifically designed for women is usually inexpensive and will give you invaluable strategies you can use to surprise, delay, neutralize, and scare off assailants. The training is also a good complement to running.
- **Don't stop and talk to strangers.** That old childhood adage still applies: Don't strike up a conversation unless you know the other person. Ignore anyone verbally harassing you. If you're being followed, get out of there fast or turn and stare at the person, to let him know you are aware of his presence and can identify him.
- **Turn an attacker in.** If you are attacked, compose yourself and memorize everything—the attacker's face, height and weight, clothes, and anything unusual such as birthmarks, scars, facial hair, and so forth. Call the police immediately, and do everything possible to catch and prosecute him.

UNIQUE PHYSICAL HEALTH ISSUES

When I first began serious running in the mid-1970s, doctors warned us that running long distances would make our breasts droop and our ovaries shrivel. When that didn't happen, the medical experts saw that regular exercise only helped women, and they said "go for it." We did, only to discover some unique conditions different from the afore-mentioned ones that can apply during training.

- **Vaginitis:** Characterized by discharge, itching, odor, and discomfort, vaginitis is caused by yeast infections, not training, but can be exacerbated by polyester fabrics that don't breathe as well as cotton and rayon. Switch to cotton training apparel and treat it with appropriate medication or consult your gynecologist.

- **Stress urinary incontinence:** Don't let this involuntary urine leakage, caused by an upsurge in abdominal and bladder pressure during exercise and coughing/sneezing, stop you. Training increases the leaks, which occur main-ly in mothers and older women, but does not worsen a preexisting condition. To lessen the flow, urinate before a training run or race and regularly do Kegel exercises (pelvic floor exercises) that can strengthen the muscles involved. A mini-pad helps, too.

- **Contraception:** Training has no effect on your contra-ceptives. Continue to use your contraceptive agent based on your needs, as normal.

- **Irregular periods (amenorrhea):** Irregular menstrual cycles are an inconvenience more common to athletically active women than sedentary women. Causes include the physical stress of training, the emotional stress of com-petition, hormonal changes, possible loss of body weight due to the increased physical activity and too-low calorie intake, or the general change in eating patterns and regi-ments. Some studies indicate that eating disorders, not exercise, are the primary causes. So, keep exercising and eating. Note: Manipulating frequent, prolonged, heavy, or unexpected menstrual periods with hormones is not recommended. Over the long term, there is no issue; normal periods usually resume once there are sufficient calories to match expenditure from training, and fertil-ity is restored to normal upon resumption of a normal menstrual cycle. As a matter of fact, after months and months of 100+ miles of running per week, I never missed a cycle.

- **Menstrual cramps:** Exercise is a boon for women who suffer from menstrual discomfort or lower abdominal pain, because it helps to alleviate symptoms. It's perfectly safe to keep training at all times during the month, even if menstrual cramps are frequent or regularly severe or debilitating. Consult your gynecologist.

ADVICE FOR MEN

With the exception of one unique anatomical issue listed here, male runners don't have any specific safety risks, as do older folks and women. But their big challenge is to keep the needs of their partners in mind in order to maintain healthy, happy, and socially enjoyable running.

- **Don't sneak up on women runners, especially single women.** Since women are rightfully paranoid, be sensitive. Also, protect yourself; if you surprise a gal, you could get maced or punched. Advertise your approach with a corny "beep-beep" or some other signal when you come within her hearing range.

- **Don't run one step ahead of any partner.** It's irritat-ing. You either wanted companionship on a run, and the benefits that come with it, or you didn't. If you don't quell the competitive instinct when your partner isn't into it, he or she may not want to run with you again. If you really want to turn up the juice, talk about it first.

- **Be encouraging with women.** Most females don't respond to men's competitive challenges as well as other men do. They do respond to camaraderie and shows of concern. So, be the nice guy that you really are.

- **Buy nipple protectors.** Yep, they exist, and they work. If you, get bloody, sandpapered nips from your polyes-ter singlet scraping you on longer runs (not a problem for bra-wearing beings), apply a thick coating of sports lube or affix these small round bandages to your nipples. Regular Band-aid strips will do the trick, too. A few carried in your pack will also take care of foot blisters.

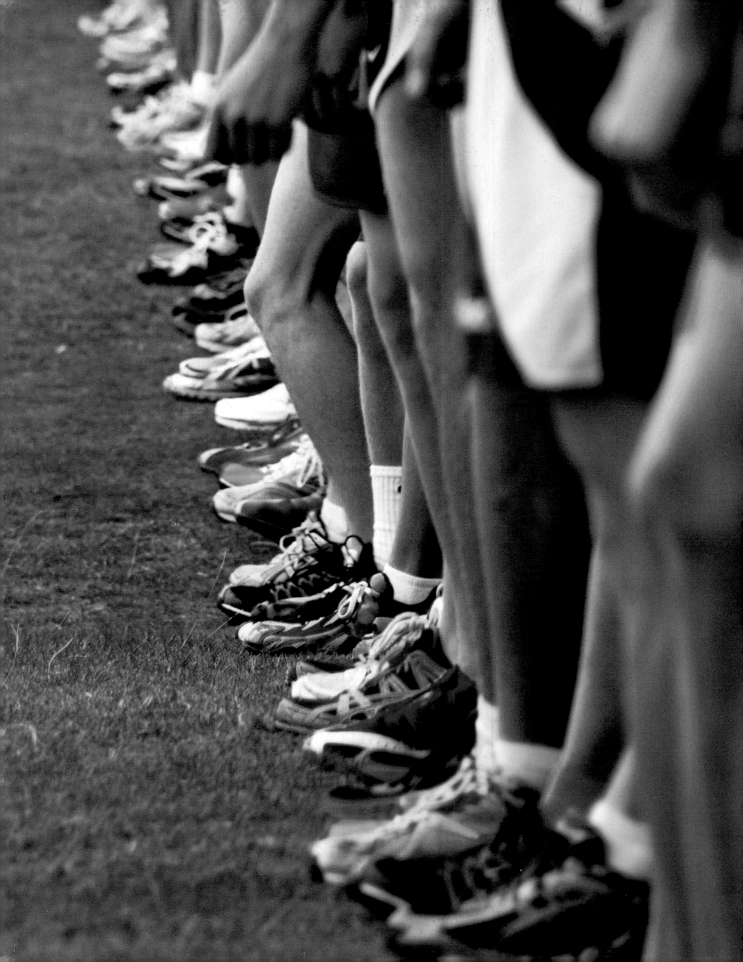

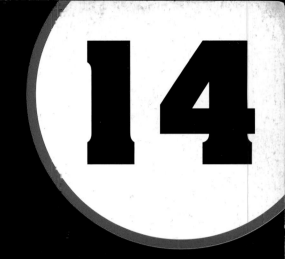

READY TO RACE
5k, 10k, HALF-MARATHON, AND
MARATHON TRAINING PLANS

FOCUSING EXCLUSIVELY ON VOLUME, VOLUME, VOLUME ... IS WRONG, WRONG, WRONG.
As we have emphasized repeatedly in this book, training for running events, whether it be
5k, 10k, half-marathon, marathon or any other distance, involves a lot more than volume.
Yes, it's true that runners love to count their miles, and love to train by running 4 miles
(6.4 km) on Monday, 5 miles (8 km) on Friday, and 8 miles (12.8 km) on Sunday. But this
common misconception—that mileage is all that matters—leads runners to overtraining,
poor performance, and injuries. Using volume alone as your training variable is not very
scientific; it neither accurately measures how much work you actually put in on a particular
training session (for example, a mile with hills is a lot more work and effort than a mile on a
level track), nor does it serve a specific purpose. If you want to really improve—that is, get
fitter, faster, and truly reach your potential—your training plan must mix and match varying levels of volume and varying levels of intensity, and (don't forget this one) accurately
measure them.

That's why, instead of the standard-issue, volume-centric training plans anyone can find all over the Web, these training plans are based around your running in specific zones—Heart Rate Training Zones—that allow you to specifically dial-in purposeful workouts that numerically quantify just how much work you are actually doing.

As you know by now, Heart Zones Training makes extensive use of your heart rate data to figure out how easy or hard your efforts should be. To do this accurately, it divides your effort range into five definable zones—blue, green, yellow, orange, and red, progressing from lowest heart rate to highest, from easiest zone to hardest. As a reminder, here is how the five zones are organized:

ZONE #	COLOR	DESCRIPTION	% OF THRESHOLD
Zone 2	GREEN	Moderate Aerobic	70-80% of Threshold
Zone 3	YELLOW	Hard Aerobic	80-90% of Threshold
Zone 4	ORANGE	Extreme Aerobic	90-100% of Threshold
Low THRESHOLD (T_1)	RED	—	100%
Zone 5a (Black Hole)	RED	Anaerobic	100-105 % of Threshold
High THRESHOLD (T_2)	RED	—	105%
Zone 5b	RED	Anaerobic Extreme	106-110% of Threshold
Zone 5c	RED	Anaerobic Insanity	110+% of Threshold

COMPILING YOUR HEART ZONES TRAINING POINTS (HZT)

Using the Heart Zones format, the various training plans here often will typically instruct you to run hard one day and easy the next, which follows the basic "Avoid the Black Hole" training strategy discovered by Dr. Steven Seiler that this book strongly advocates; this allows for the optimal challenge/recovery cycle that best increases performance.

Of course, the best way to know what Heart Zone you're in is to use a heart-rate monitor (HRM), which I strongly recommend because it is an exact measurement device and dirt-cheap (good ones start under $50).

Furthermore, using an HRM with the Heart Zones format lets you precisely and objectively quantify the workload you actually performed during your workout by using Heart Zones Training Points. As you may remember from chapter 2, calculating HZT points is simple: Multiply the number of the zone you ran in times the number of minutes in that zone. Example: 10 minutes in Zone 3 = 30 HZT Points. Enter the total in your log.

FINDING THRESHOLD WITHOUT A HEART RATE MONITOR

Naturally, trying to figure out what Heart Zone you are in is not going to be easy without a heart rate monitor. But even if you don't own or like using an HRM, you still can generally identify your basic training zones through non-monitor methods, discussed earlier in the book, that call upon you to be sensitive to the stress levels of your own body. These include perceived levels of exertion and the Foster Talk Test, the latter of which allows you to estimate the key number in any training: threshold.

Remember that threshold, as you can see visually in the accompanying color-coded chart as the 100% line, is technically a "crossover" point. It's when you crossover from a Zone 4 pace, where you get in all the O_2 you need to keep running at a comfortable pace you can maintain for hours, to a faster, more stressful Zone 5 pace, where breathing gets harder and you can't get in enough O_2 to run for more than 20 to 60 minutes, max. On the chart, you'll see that threshold is the line between Zone 4 and Zone 5. A fairly accurate way of identifying your threshold even without looking at the chart or wearing a heart-rate monitor is through the aforementioned "Talk Test." When it suddenly becomes hard to talk easily to a training partner, or recite the Pledge of Allegiance out load, you're at threshold.

In theory, once you know what threshold feels like, you can come up with a good ballpark estimate of your zones.

THE GENERAL STRATEGY: BUILD, STRENGTHEN, SHARPEN, AND TAPER FOR TOP RACE DAY PERFORMANCE

The plans outlined in the following pages will be general in nature to appeal a wide range of readers. They assume that the user will be an experienced runner, not a beginner, who therefore has some miles in his or her legs and a basic level of fitness. For this reason, the time frames the plans cover can be relatively short, reflecting what I think is a practical planning horizon for busy people in the modern world: 8 weeks for the 5k and 10k plans, 10 weeks for the half-marathon plan, and 12 weeks for the marathon plan.

Each plan will typically include 3 or 4 days of running per week, plus some cross-training, in order to assure a proper combination of workload, recovery, and variety that will improve fitness. Whatever you do, don't forget the basic principles of the Black Hole: Easy days should be easy and hard days should be hard, with hard days always followed by easy days to lock-in the gains of training.

Regardless of the target event's distance, the long-term goal of any training schedule is to progressively ramp up your fitness in a classic "periodized" manner. The three shorter-distance plans (5k, 10k, half-marathon) build you up in two major periods, or "meso-cycles," that first solidify your technique and fitness base and then enhance speed and endurance, before tapering off to keep you fresh for race day. The first meso-cycle, typically four or five weeks long, uses a lot of steady-state running to build base endurance. After a recovery week, the second four- or five-week meso-cycle builds strength and speed with hill training and intervals. Ideally, the training loads of this tried-and-true duo-phase training methodology (which is stretched into three phases, or meso-cycles, in the longer marathon program), should be carefully monitored the whole time and logged in a training diary to ensure compliance. Doing so keeps you more involved with your program, prevents overtraining, and ultimately leaves you strong, fast, fresh and at a fitness peak when you toe the start line.

GLOSSARY OF RUNS

No matter your targeted race —5k, 10, half- or full-marathon—the plans for it will make use of similar tools and terminology. We will define these here so that you can refer back to them as you work your way through the daily/weekly training plan grids.

A. TYPES OF RUNNING (AND NON-RUNNING) WORKOUTS
1. Steady Eddy

This is a steady-state run, generally used once a week, that is designed to build endurance. It can be done in any Heart Zone for any distance, but is usually in Zones 3 and 4. Start and end all Steady Eddys with an easy 5-minute warm-up in Zone 2.

2. Intervals

This is a series of relatively hard efforts, interspersed with easy recovery periods, that is designed to make you fitter and faster. An interval does not necessarily have to be an all-out, gut-busting, Zone 5 sprint; it can be at the top end of any Heart Zone.

3. Recovery Run

This is a low-intensity, low-stress easy run, typically in Zone 2 or Zone 3, that is designed to help you recuperate and rest after harder runs and intervals. A slow Steady Eddy could be a recovery run.

4. Combination Run

This is a run that uses more than one type of run during a workout — some Steady Eddy, some Intervals, for example.

5. Cross-training

This can be any athletic activity other than running, such as cycling, swimming, rowing, hiking, tennis, racquetball, and others that can allow active, non-ballistic recovery any time in any cycle.

B. BENCHMARK TRAINING TESTS
1. Observation Run

Simply go for a run at your favorite, enjoyable, standard pace, see what it feels like, and record the distance over the required time. Observe your breathing, your heart rate, your perspiration, your effort level, how fast and far you ran — and write it all down. Done during the first week of your training, it also gives you a benchmark that you will use to gauge your progress.

2. Threshold Field Test

Used during the first week of every training plan, this test helps you find the essential fitness benchmark that you will use every day: Threshold heart rate, or T_1, the heart rate upon which to establish your five Heart Zones. You cannot know where your zones limits are located, and how fast or slow to go, until you know your 100% — your threshold. In the Heart Zones system, threshold is the point at which you pass from Zone 4 to Zone 5, literally the line between the two. In overly simple terms, many people think of threshold as the point at which you begin to transition from aerobic to anaerobic metabolism.

To find your T_1 threshold, you can use the aforementioned Foster Talk test. If you run with a friend, keep talking as you increase your speed. Do not simply run as fast as you can; after a 10-minute warmup, start at a pace slower than your normal run and gradually increase your speed by 0.5 miles (0.8 km) per hour every few minutes. Constantly monitor yourself. The point at which breathing becomes difficult enough that you can no longer talk comfortably indicates that you have reached or surpassed threshold. If wearing an HRM, look at your watch and note your heart rate at threshold, your T_1 heart rate. Now, set your HRM to beep here.

Later in the training cycle, you will do a Field Test at a higher threshold level, T_2, which is the heartrate at 105% of threshold. Example: if your T_1 theshold is 150, your T_2 threshold would be 157. (Remember that the Black Hole, the area you want to stay out of as much as possible, is the area between T_1 and T_2.)

3. 1.5-mile (2.4 km) Speed Test

This 1.5-mile run, done as fast as you can in the first or second week of training, will give you another key fitness benchmark: your current aerobic running capacity. This distance, incidentally, is considered a long-enough distance to measure endurance rather than pure speed, yet short enough to not stress your body and disrupt the flow of a training plan. Systematic training can change your speed and endurance dramatically; to find out how much, the test, done as a .75-mile (1.2 km) out-and-back course or six laps around a standard quarter-mile high school track, will be repeated as one of the final workouts.

You'll perform this test by warming up for three to 10 minutes, checking your HRM, then running at your highest sustainable pace for 1.5 miles (2.4 km). Record your time and minutes per mile pace. Cooldown for 5 or 10 minutes in Zone 2.

4. "How Far Can You Go in 15?" Test

This hard, fast benchmark measures your current level of running fitness and can be repeated later to gauge improvement. After a 5-minute Zone 1 warm-up, run in Zone 4 at a constant 90% of your threshold heart rate for 15 minutes. Do 2 to 3 repeats on a treadmill for the most accurate mileage count, ending the workout with a 5 to 10-minute Zone 2 cooldown.

C. UNIQUE TRAINING WORKOUTS
1. Hold That Midpoint

Use this steady-state Zone 3 run at 85% of threshold to build upon a developed endurance base. After a 5 to 10 minute Zone 1 warm-up, fix your pace at Zone 3.5 pace for 30 to 50 minutes or 3 to 6 miles, followed by a 5 to 10 minute Zone 2 cooldown.

2. Heart Rate Ladder

This fun, challenging combination run, typically used in the second or third week, is designed to build both endurance and strength. After a 5-minute Zone 2 warm-up, you move up the "ladder" by increasing speed and intensity by 5 beats per minute every 5 minute "rung" until you reach threshold (the top of Zone 4). Then drop back down to the bottom of Zone 2 and climb the ladder again. Do two or three sets before ending the workout with a 5-minute Zone 2 cooldown.

3. Hill Repeats

Inserted into your training about half-way through the schedule after you have built a base strong enough to handle super-hard work, this high-intensity incline workout builds strength and power. It sets the stage for the speedwork to follow. After a 10-miunte Zone 2 warm-up, run hard up a hill in Zones 3 and 4 until your heart rate reaches threshold, then drop back down the hill until you recover to 70% of heart rate — and do it again and again. Rack up 5 or 10 repeats in a 20 to 45-minute period, then end the workout with a 5 to 10-minute Zone 1 cooldown. The workout can also be done on a treadmill, elliptical, or stepmill.

4. 40-Beat Zig Zag

This fun, rigorous challenge is a super speed-builder that works by pushing the body to the limit and teaching it how to recover form all-out sprints. After a 10-minute Zone 2 warmup, "kiss the ceiling" — 110% of threshold, Zone 5b. After the kiss, drop back down approximately 40 heart beats per minute to the bottom of Zone 4 (about 80% of Threshold), then blow it back up to 5b. Do this as many times possible in a 35 to 60-minute workout, closing it out on a 5 to 10-minute Zone 1 cooldown.

THE 5K TRAINING PLAN

This classic 8-week periodized training plan builds your base for two weeks, builds endurance for the next two weeks, builds strength and speed in the next two, and brings you to a peak of fitness with short, high-intensity work in week 7 before tapering for the race at the end of week 8. Of course, in keeping with the basic science of training espoused in this book, it generally avoids running two days in a row and always tries to follow a hard day with an easy day.

WEEK & TRAINING GOAL	MONDAY	TUESDAY	WEDNESDAY
Week 1: Testing & Base Building	Observation Run 30 min.	Cross-train	Threshold Field Test for 30 min
Week 2: More Base Building	1.5-Mile (2.4 km) Speed Test	Cross-train	Heart-Rate Ladder 40–50 min.
Week 3: Endurance	Steady Eddy Zone 3 30–40 min.	Hold that Midpoint (Measure time and distance) 20–30 min.	Cross-train
Week 4: More Endurance	Hill Repeats As many as possible in 45 min.	Cross-train	1.5-mile (2.4 km) Speed
Week 5: Strength	Cross-train	Steady Eddy Zone 3 1 Hour	Cross-train
Week 6: Speed Training	Interval Zone 5a Run 30–60 min.	Threshold Field Test, High (T_2) 45–50 min.	Cross-train
Week 7: Peak Training	Steady Eddy Near bottom of Zone 4 60–90 min.	Cross-train	Long Intervals 35–60 min.
Week 8: Taper & Race	Half 40-beat ZigZag	Steady Eddy Near bottom of Zone 4 30-45 min.	Cross-train

THURSDAY	FRIDAY	SATURDAY	SUNDAY	LOAD IN HZT POINTS
Zone 3 Steady Eddy 40 min.	Cross-train	Steady Eddy Zone 3 45 min.	Rest Day Stretch	450 Points
Cross-train	Steady Eddy Zone 3 30–45 min.	"How Far Can You Go in 15?" Test	Rest Day Stretch	350–650 Points
Threshold Field Test 40-45 min.	Cross-train	Steady Eddy Zone 3 40 min.	Rest Day Stretch	400–710 Points
Steady Eddy Zone 3 45 min.	Cross-train	Hill Repeats. As many as possible in 50 min.	Rest Day Stretch	455–750 Points
Hill Repeats. As many as possible in one hour	Cross-train	Steady Eddy Zone 3.5 1 Hour	Rest Day Stretch	500–800 Points
Intervals—Extra long. Do them 3-off, 1-on 40–50 min.	Cross-train	40-beat Zig Zag 40 min.	Rest Day Stretch	550–850 Points
Cross-train	Hill Repeats 0–50 min.	Cross-train	Rest Day Stretch	600–900 Points
Combo Run. 20 min., include Zone 3 steady running and Zone 4 intervals	Rest Day Stretch	The Race	Rest Day Stretch	300–450 Points

THE 10K TRAINING PLAN

The 10k plan features an 8-week periodized game plan like that of the 5k plan—two weeks each of base building, endurance, and strength and speed, with a high-intensity push to a fitness peak week 7 and a taper to race day in week 8—but factors in longer distances on the Steady Eddy and other runs. For example, "How Far Can You Go in 15?" changes to "How Far Can You go in 25?"

WEEK & TRAINING GOAL	MONDAY	TUESDAY	WEDNESDAY
Week 1: Testing & Base Building	Observation Run 30 min.	Cross-train	Threshold Field Test for 30 min.
Week 2: More Base Building	1.5-Mile (2.4 km) Speed Test, followed by Steady Eddy 75% of threshold for 15-30 min.	Cross-train	Heart-Rate Ladder 40–50 min.
Week 3: Endurance	Steady Eddy Zone 3 50–70 min.	Stretch	Hold That Midpoint (Measure time and distance) 20–30 min.
Week 4: More Endurance	Cross-train	Hill Repeats. As many as possible in 45 min.	Stretch
Week 5: Strength	1.5-mile (2.4 km) Speed + Steady Eddy Zone 3 45 min.	Hill Repeats. As many as possible in 1 Hour	Cross-train
Week 6: Speed Training	Threshold Field Test, High (T_2) 45–50 min.	Cross-train	Intervals—Extra long. Do them 3-off, 1-on For 1 Hour
Week 7: Peak Training	Steady Eddy Top of Zone 4 60-90 min.	Cross-train	Long Intervals 50–80 min.
Week 8: Taper & Race	Half 40-beat ZigZag	Steady Eddy Near bottom of Zone 4 40-60 min.	Cross-train

THURSDAY	FRIDAY	SATURDAY	SUNDAY	LOAD IN HZT POINTS
Stretch Day- stretching, yoga, flexibility	Cross-train	Steady Eddy Midpoint of Zone 4 36-70 min	Rest Day Stretch	400-630 Points
Cross-train	Steady Eddy Zone 3 40–65 min.	"How Far Can You Go in 25?" Test	Rest Day Stretch	350–650 Points
Cross-train	Threshold Field Test 40-45 min.	Rest Day Stretch	Long Slow Distance Steady Eddy Zone 3 1 Hour	400–710 Points
Steady Eddy Zone 4 1 Hour	Cross-train	"How Far Can You Go in 25?" Test	Rest Day Stretch	490–780 Points
Steady Eddy Zone 3.5 1.25 Hours	Cross-train	Hill Repeats. As many as possible in 1 Hour	Rest Day Stretch	550–870 Points
Cross-train	40-beat Zig Zag 1.25 hrs	Steady Eddy Bottom of Zone 4 1 Hour	Rest Day Stretch	570–890 Points
Cross-train	Hill Repeats 1 Hour	"How Far Can You Go in 25?" Test	Rest Day Stretch	630–950 Points
Combo Run 30 min., include Zone 3 steady running and Zone 4 intervals	Rest Day Stretch	The Race	Rest Day Stretch	360–510 Points

THE HALF-MARATHON TRAINING PLAN

The training plan for a half-marathon increases to a 10-week periodized schedule. After building up a training load from 700 to 1050 HZT points for four weeks, with your long weekly run rising in length from 5 miles (8 km) to 7 miles (11.2 km), this plan lets you rest and recover with a 600-point "off-load" week after a month. As speed and strength

WEEK & TRAINING GOAL	MONDAY	TUESDAY	WEDNESDAY
Week 1: **Base Building**	Steady Eddy Zone 3 15-30 min.	Cross-train	*Day Off*
Week 2: **Base Buildin**	1.5-mile Speed Test + Steady Eddy Zone 3 midpoint 10-30 min.	Cross-train	Heart Rate Ladder 15-30 min.
Week 3: **Endur ance**	Heart Rate Ladder 20-40 min.	Cross-train	Hill Repeats 20-45 min.
Week 4: **Endurance**	40-Beat ZigZag 35-60 min.	Cross-train	Steady Eddy Low Zone 4 40-60 min.
Week 5: **Off Load Recovery Week**	Long Walk and Stretching	Steady Eddy Zones 2-4 20-40 min.	Cross-train
Week 6: Strength	Intervals 5 min. repeats at 100% of threshold, 2-min. rest 35-70 min.	Cross-train	1.5-mile Speed Test + Steady Eddy Zone 3.5 30-60 min.
Week 7: Speed	Cross-train	Intervals 3 min. Fast 1 min. Slow Zone 5b & Zone 3 30-40 min.	Steady Eddy Zone 3 40-75 min.
Week 8: Power	Cross-train	Hill Repeats 40-60 min.	Steady Eddy Zone 4.5 45-80 min.
Week 9: **Peak**	Cross-train	Intervals 2x10 min. Zone 4 85% for 10 min. and 95% for 10 min. repeat 4x, 7-9 miles 90-100 min.	Steady Eddy High Zone 4 50-85 min.
Week 10: **Taper and Race**	15 min. each in Zones 3-4 at 80, 90, 95, 100% of threshold 50 min. total	Cross-train	"Test-drive" the pace. Do 1 mile at race pace with 3 min. rest. Repeat for 35-40 min.

work pick up after the break in week 6, the training load rises to a peak of 1400 HZT points in week 9 with a maximum run of 11 miles before dropping to 400 HZT points and a 5-miler on the week 10 on the taper for race-day.

Note: All workout times listed below do not include 5-to 10-minute warm-up and cool-down.

THURSDAY	FRIDAY	SATURDAY	SUNDAY	LOAD IN HZT POINTS
Threshold Field Test	Cross-train	Observation Run	Cross-train	300-400 Points
Day Off	"How Far Can You Go in 15?"	Cross-train	Combo Run Zone 3 Alternate 80% and 90% of threshold every 5 min. 30-50 min.	450 Points
Hold That Midpoint Zone 3.5 30-50 min.	Cross-train	Un-Steady Eddy Zones 3, 4 Alternate intervals at 80, 85, 90% of threshold 36-60 min.	Cross-train	590 Points
Cross-train	Hill Repeats 30-50 min.	Cross-train	Steady Eddy High Zone 4 40-75 min.	840 Points
Steady Eddy Zones 2-4 20-40 min.	Read a Book	Steady Eddy Zones 1-3 25-45 min.	Go Shopping	300-400 Points
Cross-train	Hill Repeats 30-50 min.	Cross-train	Race Pace Intervals 10-min. intervals at race pace w/ 2-min. rest 40-60 min.	910 Points
Cross-train	Hill Repeats 35-55 min.	Indoor Cross-train Zone 4 Tread, ellip., bike, stairs 12 min. each 48 min.	Run Race Pace Zone 4	1,130 Points
Cross-train	Track Intervals Zones 4-5 5x400 yd 1x800 yd 30-40 min	Cross-train	10-mile Run Pace Zone 4	1,200 Points
Cross-train	Hill Repeats Zones 3-5 Ascend to 95-105% of threshold Repeat 7-10x 35-40 min.	Cross-train	11-mile Run Zone 4	1,415 Points
Day off-optional with cross-training	Steady Eddy Zones 3-4 25-35 min.	Complete Rest Day	The race	405 Points + the race

THE MARATHON TRAINING PLAN

The 12-week marathon plan is similar to the half-marathon program, with several upgrades: It starts with longer times and higher mileage, changes the "How Far Can You Run in 15?" test to 25 minutes, and goes from two 5-week phases to three 4-week phases.

Phase 1, as with the 5k, 10k, and half-marathon training plans, focuses on base-building and endurance, specifically improving stamina and aerobic capacity as you progressively increase the training load. The goal of the Phase 2 is to improve sport-specific muscle strength (e.g., hill runs),

WEEK & TRAINING GOAL	MONDAY	TUESDAY	WEDNESDAY
Phase 1			
Week 1: Base Building	Steady Eddy Zone 3 25–45 min.	Cross-train	Threshold Field Test
Week 2: Base Building	1.5 mile Speed Test + Steady Eddy Zone 3.5 20–45 min	Cross-train	Heart Rate Ladder 30–45 min.
Week 3: Endurance	Cross-train	Heart Rate Ladder 30–60 min.	Cross-train
Week 4: Endurance	40-Beat ZigZag 45–80 min.	Cross-train	Intervals 60 min.
Phase 2			
Week 5: Strength	Hill Repeats 4–5 reps 45 min.	Steady Eddy Zone 3 55 min.	Cross-train
Week 6: Strength	Cross-train	Steady Eddy Zone 3 45 min.	Hill Repeats 4–5 reps 45 min.
Week 7: Recovery	Cross-train	Steady Eddy Zone 3 55 min.	Hill Repeats 2–3 reps 25 min.
Week 8 : Speed	Cross-train	Intervals Zone 5 30 min.	Hill Repeats 6–10 reps 60 min.

increase average weekly mileage, and get faster with interval training and combination runs. Phase 3 raises your fitness and speed to a peak by combining hill training, speed training, and endurance training, adding weekly time trials to give you an accurate estimate of the race pace and heart rate percentage you'll be using on marathon race day.

Note: All workout times listed below do not include 5- to 10-minute warm-up and cool-down.

THURSDAY	FRIDAY	SATURDAY	SUNDAY	LOAD IN HZT POINTS
Phase 1				
Cross-train	Steady Eddy Zone 4 35 min.	Cross-train	Steady Eddy Zone 3 60 min	445 Points
Cross-train	"How Far Can You Go in 25?"	Cross-train	Steady Eddy Zone 3 70 min.	565 Points
Hold That Midpoint Zone 3.5 45 min.	Cross-train	Steady Eddy Zone 3 80 min.	Cross-train Zone 4 45 min.	705 Points
Steady Eddy Zone 4 50 min.	Rest Day	Combination Zone 3 90 min.	Steady Eddy High Zone 4 50–90 min. (or 8 miles)	830 Points
Phase 2				
Intervals Zone 4 40 min.	Rest Day	Intervals Zone 5b 30 Min.	Steady Eddy Zone 3.5 60–100 min. (or 10 miles)	1,055 Points
Steady Eddy Zone 4 40 min.	Rest Day	Combination Zone 3 for 15 Zone 5b for 15–30 min.	Steady Eddy Zone 3.5 80–120 min. (or 13 miles)	1,190 Points
Steady Eddy Zone 3 40 min.	Rest Day	Hill Repeats 2–3 reps 35 min.	Steady Eddy Zone 3.5 90–130 min. (or 15 miles)	425 Points
Steady Eddy Zone 4 50 min.	Rest Day	Combination Zone 3 for 15 Zone 5b for 15–30 min.	Steady Eddy Zone 3.5 100–140 min. (or 17 miles)	1,350 Points

WEEK & TRAINING GOAL	MONDAY	TUESDAY	WEDNESDAY
Phase 3			
Week 9: Speed	Cross-train	Intervals 20 min Zone 5b 20 min Zone 3	Steady Eddy recovery workout Zone 3 60 min.
Week10: Power	Cross-train	Intervals 20 min. Zone 5b 20 min. Zone 3 60 min.	Cross-train
Week 11: Peak	Cross-train	20 min. Zone 5b 20 min. Zone 3	Hill Repeats 4–5 reps 45 min.
Week 12: Taper and Race	Rest Day	Steady Eddy Zone 3 40 min.	Steady Eddy Zone 4 60 min.

MILES TO KILOMETERS CONVERSION CHART

MILES	KILOMETERS	MILES	KILOMETERS
1	1.60	14	22.53
2	3.21	15	24.14
3	4.82	16	25.74
4	6.43	17	27.35
5	8.04	18	28.96
6	9.65	19	30.57
7	11.26	20	32.18
8	12.87	21	33.79
9	14.48	22	35.40
10	16.09	23	37.01
11	17.70	24	38.62
12	19.31	25	40.23
13	20.92	26	41.84

THURSDAY	FRIDAY	SATURDAY	SUNDAY	LOAD IN HZT POINTS
Phase 3				
Hill Repeats 6–10 reps 70 min.	Rest Day	Combo Zone 3, 4 70 min.	Steady Eddy Zone 4 120–160 min. (or 18 miles)	1,620 Points
Steady Eddy Time trial: 60 min. at marathon pace	Hill Repeats 4-5 reps. 40 min.	Cross-train	Steady Eddy Zone 4 120–160 min. (or 20 miles)	1,720 Points
Recovery 20 min. Zone 5b 20 min Zone 3	Rest Day	Recovery Zone 4 70 min.	Steady Eddy Zone 4 100–120 min. (or 13 miles)	1,620 Points
Rest Day	Steady Eddy Zone 4 40 min.	Attend the Marathon Expo	The Marathon	360 Points + your marathon points

PHOTO CREDITS

ABOUT THE AUTHORS

SALLY EDWARDS is a former master's world record holder in the Ironman Triathlon, a 1984 Olympic marathoner trials finisher as well as a world record holder in the Iditashoe 100-Mile Snowshoe Race. She has competed in some of the hardest races on the planet, including the Western States 100-Mile Run which she won. A leader in the field of fitness training, Sally holds a master's in exercise physiology and is the creator and CEO of the Heart Zones Training System, which uses heart rate data and cardiac training ranges to enhance athletic performance. A founder of the sport of triathlon (and a Triathlon Hall of Fame inductee), most of Sally's recent races have been performed in her role as the national spokeswoman for the Danskin Triathlon Series.

CARL FOSTER PH.D., FACSM, is the former president of the American College of Sports Medicine. He is a professor of exercise and sport science at the University of Wisconsin–La Crosse and director of the Human Performance Laboratory at UW–L. Carl is a former associate editor-in-chief of *Medicine and Science in Sports and Exercise,* and a co-editor of American College of Sports Medicine's *Health/Fitness Facility Standards and Guidelines.* His distinguished professional career and accomplishments have produced over 250 scientific papers, book chapters, and longer works.

ROY M. WALLACK is a longtime writer, editor, and author specializing in fitness training, gear, and adventure travel. A fitness columnist for the *Los Angeles Times,* he is the former editor of *Triathlete* and *Bicycle Guide* magazines, and a contributor to a variety of magazines, including *Outside, Men's Journal, Runner's World, Muscle & Fitness, Playboy, Competitor, Consumer's Digest, Bicycling, Mountain Bike,* and others. His books include *Run for Life: The Breakthrough Plan for Fast Times, Fewer Injuries, and Spectacular Lifelong Fitness* (2009), *Bike for Life: How to Ride to 100* (2005), and *The Traveling Cyclist: 20 Worldwide Tours of Discovery* (1991). A frequent participant in some of the world's toughest endurance events, including the Badwater Ultramarathon, the Eco-Challenge, the 750-mile Paris-Brest-Paris randonee, and the TransAlp Challenge, he was inducted into the 24 Hours of Adrenaline Solo Hall of Fame in 2008 and finished second in the World Fitness Championship in 2004.

INDEX

overuse, 195

    preventing, 196–197

in-line skating, 54

input-output curves, 98

insole, 169

intensity, 104–107

internal goals, 121, 123

intervals, 107–108, 204

Ironman World Series, 136

J

Jansen, Elizabeth, 158

Jeans, Beth, 105

jogging stroller, 170

Johnson, Brooks, 148

jumping rope, 56

K

Klark, Craig, 146

Klotkowski, Stan, 113

L

lace locks, 172

lactate response, 104–105

lactate threshold, 25, 29

Lieberman, Daniel, 11, 141, 143, 150–151

light training days, 43–44

long-term goals, 121, 123

lube, 173

Lydiard, Arthur, 46, 96

M

Map My Run, 78

marathon training plan, 212–213

maximum heart rate, 28, 104

McDonald, Ted, 146

McDougall, Christopher, 141, 143

men, 199

menstrual cramps, 199

metabolic load, 35

metabolism, 132, 186

midsole, 168

mission statement, 123–129

training strain, 113

training volume, 100–103

treadmills, 84–87, 169

triceps stretch, 72

TRIMPS (training impulse), 12, 106, 108–110

tripping, 196

U

underpronation, 161

UpBeat Workouts, 170

upper, 168

V

vaginitis, 199

variability training, 43–44

varying meso cycle, 112

ventilatory response, 104–105

ventilatory threshold, 28

visibility, 77

vitamin D, 186

VO_2 max, 28, 52, 98, 104

volume multipliers, 102

W

Wallack, Roy M., 147

warming up, 73, 133

water, 134, 188–191

wear test, 161–163

weight loss, 186–188

weight training, 13, 57–61

Wherry, Erica, 106

Williams, Keith, 150

Williams' flexion hamstring stretch, 71

women, 196, 197–199

workouts, recovery from, 42–43

wrist-top devices, 170

Y

Young, Ken, 100

Z